COMPLEMENTARY MEDICINE
AND THE EUROPEAN COMMUNITY

Edited by
George Lewith MA MRCP MRGCP
and David Aldridge PhD

Index compiled by
Mary Toase ALA

SAFFRON WALDEN
THE C.W. DANIEL COMPANY LIMITED

First published in book form
in Great Britain
by The C.W. Daniel Company Ltd
1 Church Path, Saffron Walden, Essex CB10 1JP, England

ISBN 0 85207 234 1

Design and Production in association
with Book Production Consultants, Cambridge, England.

Typeset by Anglia Photoset, Colchester
Printed and bound in England by St Edmundsbury Press,
Bury St Edmunds, Suffolk.

COMPLEMENTARY MEDICINE
AND THE EUROPEAN COMMUNITY

THE BRITISH SCHOOL OF OSTEOPATHY
1-4 SUFFOLK ST., LONDON. SW1Y 4HG
TEL. 01 - 930 9254-8

Contents

Introduction

In this collection of review papers we have looked at the major areas of interest within the European Economic Community pertaining to complementary medicine.

The first chapter by Harald Gaier analyses in some detail the legal position of complementary practitioners within the European Community and how this will ultimately effect training and practice in all the member states. Many of the English colleges have already acted on these proposals. Fully fledged degree courses are now set up and running at the British School of Osteopathy and the Anglo-European College of Chiropractic. A number of the other colleges are now following this path by attempting to upgrade their courses while simultaneously getting recognition from the Committee for National Academic Awards.

We also have reports from individual countries, produced initially for the EEC Conference on Complementary Medicine in June 1989. This information provides much hitherto unpublished data about what is actually happening within the various members states of the Community, both from the point of view of patient use and government legislation. A knowledge of what is taking place 'on the ground' is essential if we are to make coherent decisions about future health care provision, both within the field of complementary medicine and on a more macro scale with respect to both National and Community legislation. Such massive use of the complementary therapies should also provide all of us with more impetus to research the clinical application and basic mechanisms involved.

The final chapter by Harald Gaier outlines the legislative confusion and pitfalls pertaining to the manufacture and licensing of natural remedies. The European Community clearly has a long road to travel before such legislation is uniformly accepted throughout the member states.

We believe this book provides a unique insight into complementary medicine with a European perspective and hope that it will stimulate further thought, a better quality of care, and, above all else, more research into this field of endeavour. The R.C.C.M. have taken on board a national responsibility for coordinating and directing research, and this publication should be seen as part of its efforts within this broad general field.

George Lewith,
Centre for the Study of
Complementary Medicine,
51 Bedford Place,
Southampton.

David Aldridge,
Medical Faculty
Universität Witten-Herdecke,
Beckweg 4,
D 5804 Herdecke, (Ruhr)
Germany

1990

CHAPTER 1

Reveille for biocentric medicine

Harald Gaier

Summary
Since writing on the subject of implementing an educational strategy for Biocentric Medicine[1], a situation has arisen that has taken much of the initiative out of the hands of those who wish to chart the future course for Biocentric Medicine. The fresh circumstances and their implications are discussed and concrete proposals made.

Introduction
In Biocentric medical circles there are several unresolved contentious issues.

1. The desire for some form of inspired and reflective tertiary education programme that competes equally with orthodoxy, while remaining independent of it.

2. The apprehension that the EC secretly plans to extinguish the Biocentric movement, although the EC has publicly acknowledged the independent position in society this form of medicine rightfully enjoys[2].

3. The widespread belief that there can never be an adequate academic course to teach natural ability.

4. The aim to establish ethical standards that will also conform to four consumer norms which are emerging for Biocentric health care services[3], namely:

a) full information disclosure at all levels concerning practice, equipment, medicines, fees, anticipated duration of treatment, etc;
b) verification of individual professional competence by an officially accredited institution;
c) full compliance by all practitioners and therapists (see footnote † below) with the new British Education Reform Act;
d) Practitioner/therapist accountability and ready accessibility to means of redress for any aggrieved party.

5. The apprehension at the prospect of a diminishing number of options left for self-determination by Biocentric Medicine, whilst the absence of self-regulation is seen to lead to the need for restrictions being imposed.

6. The misgivings about disunity in the Biocentric leadership, one consequence of which is that the Working Party on Alternative and Complementary Medicine (WoPACM), the Council for Complementary and Alternative Medicine (CCAM) and the Institute for Complementary Medicine (ICM) have lost the political initiative they may once have enjoyed. As a result of this the Government remains unable to make firm commitments to any of the representative bodies because none of them is fully representative.

---

† A full professional discipline is a complete, self-contained medical system such as chiropractic, homoeopathy, naturopathy, osteopathy, phytotherapy or Oriental medicine; whereas a therapy is an adjunctive treatment modality that has no pretentions to being a complete medical system, e.g. aromatherapy, reflexology, shiatsu, hypnotherapy, etc. The professional engaged in the former is correctly referred to as a practitioner, the professional engaged in the latter as a therapist.

7. The pride in the positive developments in the following two important areas:-

(i) A research project of some importance on *alternative health care* has been commenced at Sheffield University's Department of Community Medicine; and the Research Council for Complementary Medicine (RCCM) together with the UK Medical Research Council (MRC) have jointly funded a post at Glasgow University to study research methodology within the paradigm of Biocentric Medicine. Both these developments are seen as very constructive. Involving, as they do, the orthodox establishment, Biocentric ideas or therapeutic approaches may, in future, not easily be dismissed simply through lack of formalized evidence.

(ii) The planned introduction, or existence, of formal academic courses at five recognized Universities, Polytechnics or equivalent places of tertiary education (see *The Consequences 4/ and 7/* below).

8. The ambivalent attitude to the natural tensions emanating from two other poles of a tripolarity, comprising Biocentric Medicine, Government and orthodox. This net of threeway tension maintains the fluctuating equilibrium between differences in the cultural potential in medicine, as it has always done. Between the other two poles a similar state of delicately balanced tension also exists (see *The Prospects Ad 8/* below). Those other two forces, relative to the Biocentric pole, are:

(i) Governments of EC Member States, that are generating very strong socio-political pressures, principally away from emphasis on disease treatment only, towards a greater role for preventive approaches; and

(ii) the orthodox medical associations, as well as the vested pharmaceutical interests, that are generating powerful pressures to assimilate into orthodoxy's therapeutic maw those Biocentric medical methods latterly perceived to be successful (e.g. as happened with naturopathic diets and exercise therapy for longevity), or simply to attempt to discredit such methods.

9. A sense of looming economic insecurity within the rank and file of the Biocentric movement, engendered by two unsettling possibilities:
(i) The destabilizing effect, should Biocentric Medicine become the refuge for substantial numbers of registered nurses, orthodox UK doctors and paramedics, who could be displaced from their present positions in the foreseeable future as casualties of the State's medical cost containment policies.
(ii) The start of an indefinite period of unrestrictable influx into the UK of many jobless orthodox medical practioners from elsewhere in Europe.

10. A profoundly felt concern about the future of the 'customary British way' that has nurtured the Biocentric medical system here, almost like a living organism, which enabled it to spawn the evolution of the many varied practices under Common Law. The concern is that this 'customary British way' will simply be extinguished by the superimposition of an outlandish EC-inspired regimentation.
Into this relatively predictable setting a new factor has suddenly been introduced that is sure to create a significant upheaval.

The directive from the EC
On the 24th January 1989 the *Official Journal of the European Communities* (No L 19/16–23) published an important Council Directive (89/48/EC) addressed to Member States. This Directive had been promulgated one month earlier by the EC in Brussels. It is binding upon Member States and lays down the European Communities'

system for the recognition of higher education diplomas (meaning 'degrees' in Great Britain and Eire) awarded on completion of professional education and training of at least three years' duration. It is clear that this mandatory Directive will affect all practitioners of Biocentric Medicine.

A condensed interpretative rendering of this Directive, and of its imminent consequences relative to the Biocentric medical field, follows here:

If the various Biocentric Medicine disciplines are able to organize themselves as true professions, insisting on at least three years' full-time study at a tertiary level and are able to attain Governmental recognition for this, those so qualified will be entitled to practise their profession throughout the community, regardless of local (national) qualification requirements. Additionally, each national area may impose local practice-aptitude requirements (e.g. examination of an otherwise well-qualified British naturopath settled in France, on French terminology and medico-legal questions). All Member States (therefore also Eire and the UK) must have taken all the measures necessary by not later than the 3rd January 1991 for the facilitation and implementation of this mandatory Directive. This means all the courses and the recognition of degree status, and the like, will have had to be finalised between now and the end of next year. The Directive would allow for each Biocentric discipline to go its separate way on this (i.e. each with its own 3, 4 or 5 year degree course), or all these disciplines, or some of them, could combine to recognize a course of study as satisfying the requirements of all, subject, of course, to any additional period of internship or clinical experience, as would have to have been laid down by then too.

The consequences
Certain issues immediately seem to emerge from this.

1. To vacillate over the provision of Biocentric medical education would swiftly leave ever fewer options open. Although this event ought only to affect itinerant practitioners and therapists (*see footnote* page 41) in the EC, and not those who are sedentary in the United Kingdom and in Eire, it would be impractical to have one set of educational standards for the one type of practitioner and another for the second. This development will not stop Biocentric practice in the British Isles now, but it may in the foreseeable future. It may come about by stealth, by the piecemeal curtailment of a freedom now enjoyed (briefly discussed previously in *Complementary Medical Research*[1]). It seems quite clear that the standards as applicable to the whole of the EC will, by law, also apply to the educational standards to be implemented in Great Britain and in Eire before 4th January 1991.

2. What took place is seemingly a compromise between the French and German positions on the troubling question of formal education in Biocentric medicine.

3. It appears from public utterances prior to the publication of this EC Directive that the ICM, CCAM and WoPACM and others were all unaware of the preparation of the Directive. It seems likely that it was the Department of Trade and Industry which was involved in the draft stages of this Directive. The Department of Health would have been only marginally informed. Therefore, non-governmental parties like the ICM, CCAM, WoPACM, etc would not have been consulted at all. Yet they might well have been, had they been in a position to present a unified front.

4. It seems, too, that universities which offer courses in subjects related to Biocentric Medicine in the UK were unprepared for the implications of this Directive.

The *Complementary Health Studies* now available through the University of Exeter seem to lack the proper content. The syllabus obviously needed to undergo major modification and a full curriculum required to be developed. In a lengthy, detailed application to the University's Faculty Board, application to run a post-graduate degree programme was made at the beginning of this year designed to lead to a BPhil, MPhil and ultimately to a PhD degree. This application was supported by the CCAM, but it seems that at the time it was made, no knowledge of the impending Directive as in the applicants' minds, because the BPhil is a two-year part-time course only. Nonetheless, this course is a visionary first step. It foresaw the need to train the qualified nurses and paramedics, perhaps even some pharmacists.

Once trained, these are widely acknowledged to be very competent practitioners or therapists in Biocentric Medicine. What is required is an accreditation formula for the existing practitioners' preceding studies and some major adjustment of the course content, to cover the teaching of 'practice and practicalities' in Biocentric Medicine, rather than its present emphasis on theory and philosophical aspects. Given this, the BPhil degree, or in default thereof, the longer MPhil course, may yet be destined to become the standard degree, as both have now obtained faculty approval.

On the other hand, ICM's 18-month diploma course to be referred to as *Biological Foundations of Health,* now being planned (subject to funding) by the Department of Biology at the Open University, whilst also commendable, shows no foreknowledge either, because the course as envisaged is much too short to be able to qualify. It would require very major adjustments to be made. Another course in *Complementary Medicine* has now also been included in Sheffield Polytechnics' Health Sciences degree. This one course alone, however, will probably be assessed as insufficient to meet the EC-enacted requirement for qualification to practise Biocentric Medicine.

As things stand at present the only courses that would fully qualify are the four-year BSc courses in Osteopathy and Chiropractic, both of which have attained validation from the Council for National Academic Awards (CNAA). One is offered by the British School of Osteopathy, the other at the Anglo-European College of Chiropractic in Bournemouth. It seems likely that fully degree status (though not through the CNAA) will in due time be accorded also to the existing course that is offered by the British College of Naturopathy and Osteopathy (BCNO) in London, possibly by way of an affiliation to a university. That should be positively welcomed, since the BCNO's four year course offers all-round Biocentric medical education of a high calibre with a strong grounding in orthodox diagnostics (*see footnote* below†). A three year segment of the

---

† In the BCNO syllabus, 5494 hours are allotted to (subjects listed alphabetically with hours in parenthesis): anamnestic evaluation and auscultation (60); anatomy and locomotor physiology (270); biology (54); chemistry (30); clinical diagnostic assessment (1073); clinical dietetics (90); diagnosis (180); laboratory techniques (90); practice and theory of natural therapeutics (90); neuro-muscular techniques (36); nutrition (180); obstetrics and gynaecology (70); orthopaedics and traumatology (126); applied orthopaedics/clinical syndromes (36); osteopathy/techniques (1296); osteopathy/clinical assessment and applied spinal mechanics (1073); paediatrics (70); pathology (90); pharmacology (40); psychology (90); psychosomatics (90); soft-tissue techniques (90); visceral physiology (180); x-ray diagnosis and related techniques (90).

BCNO's course could become the universal foundation for all Biocentric medical education in the UK, with a choice of studies of other disciplines modularly suffixed from year four (e.g. for non-osteopathic and non-chiropractic students: acupuncture, homoeopathy, phytotherapy etc, appended with the osteopathic component concurrently reduced). After all, the BCNO has the distinction of having consistently produced some of the most outstanding practitioners ever since its first graduation in 1946.

5. Since the Directive of the European Communities stipulates that only "evidence of [such] formal qualification ... awarded by a competent authority in a Member State" can be recognized, it means that, say, a naturopathic or a chiropractic qualification from the USA, or an osteopathic degree from Australia, New Zealand or South Africa puts its holder, *prima facie*, in the category of the unqualified. But such practitioners may yet qualify, if they are able to show that their subsequent training (though the basic studies were completed outside the EC) was "received mainly in the Community" and that, moreover, each also "has three years' professional experience certified by the Member State which recognizes a third-country diploma, certificate or other evidence of formal qualifications".

6. Should uncertainty in the area of Biocentric medical education persist in the British Isles, an option open to practitioners who may be put in the position of having to change their domicile to another EC country, would be to take the recognized German course in the FRG for the Heilpraktikerschaft. With that they could practise legally, say, in the south of France, or anywhere else in the EC. It would be heartening, though, to have Great Britain also offer this possibility to nationals of other EC countries, where this is unavailable.

7. Article 3 of the Directive speaks, very explicitly, of "evidence of one or more formal qualifications ... which have prepared the holder for the pursuit of his profession". The question that arises is whether, for instance, an orthodox medical degree can be said to qualify the holder to practice, say, chiropractic; or, for that matter, homoeopathy, or any other Biocentric medical discipline, competently.

Since the French and the Germans are thought to be a major influence in the drafting of this directive, it is relevant to look at what training is obligatory there for fully qualified orthodox medical practitioners. In France four medical schools train 1000 registered doctors per year in established 3 year post-graduate courses in acupuncture, homoeopathy or phytotherapy, which eventually leads to the bestowal of the status of 'Specialist'. Anything less, though this is available too, is certainly considered as an inadequate qualification. In the FRG orthodox medical practitioners who wish to employ Biocentric Medical methods must undergo the normal training in the accredited Heilpraktiker colleges. They are granted a State licence after passing examinations.

Quite clearly, the Directive is designed to exclude the inappropriately qualified from practising so that, for instance, a British-qualified acupuncturist cannot set him/herself up as an osteopath. This, of course, raises a further issue. Can any practitioner who may be permitted to practise the discipline in which qualification was obtained, perform any action pertaining to another's profession? Will a British orthodox medical practitioner, without any formal three-year training, be entitled to manipulate or prescribe homoeopathically or undertake, say, hydrotherapy, on a patient? Will a qualified acupuncturist be able to use tuina techniques (akin to osteopathy) even if they did not form part of the formal training received? What of the British Faculty of Homoeopathy's standard introductory course for orthodox practitioners, which consists of a mere four days – hardly long enough to learn the names of the more basic three hundred or so homoeopathic remedies? Or even the full six-months' course offered there? Can they be said to prepare the certificate holder for the pursuit of the homoeopathic profession?

By contrast, the British Postgraduate Medical Federation seemed mindful of this problem. Commendably, they are setting up a one-year modular course in *Holistic Medicine* for orthodox practitioners and for healthcare professionals from the orthodox camp. The length of this course, taken together with their previous training, might certainly be adequate for practising Holistic Medicine. But how would chartered physiotherapists and registered nurses, without any further training, be assessed; who, alienated through politically-induced economic circumstances, may now wish to qualify for practising Biocentric Medicine? Under which circumstances, if at all, would a 2-year part-time BPhil degree from Exeter University be considered sufficient to satisfy the EC Directive?

Plainly, a controlling organ, with full statutory powers to regulate, is needed to be established as a matter of the utomost urgency. Surely this is a more reasonable solution, when compared with the arduous and costly alternative of establishing it through Case Law by testing such questions in the Civil Courts.

8. Although the United Kingdom could, theoretically, have veoted this mandatory Directive because it concerns professional qualifications, it has decided not to do so.

The whole issue of Biocentric medical education and its consequences need to be thought through and tackled without delay in the light of this development. Probably its most dire need of a decision is the area concerning professional unity. It is clear, too, that it is impossible on economic grounds, if on no other, for each professional discipline and each therapy (*see footnote* page 10) to have its own degree course. Therefore, it may simply have to be a jointly approved curriculum (for example, the BCNO's) for a large segment encompassing many professions. Or, perhaps, the division as outlined previously[1], should be adopted as the most feasible, after all. This division between the *medicinal* and the *physical* branches of Biocentric medicine, coincides with what Thomas has termed the *soft* and *hard* practices[4].

Another alternative may be the Electronic (computerized) audio-visual) Academy offering a broad selection through a Biocentric Educational network proposed below (under *The Prospects Ad 7/(ii)*). Yet to achieve any such rationalization presupposes absolute professional unity now. If that cannot be arrived at, Biocentric medical education is in imminent danger of being arrogated (for a very long time to come) by other who do not really wish to see it succeed.

The recent fate of two very strong branches of Biocentric Medicine in the USA (Homoeopathy and osteopathy) that succumbed to assimilation into orthodoxy should be a salutary warning. MacEoin[5] points out that homoeopathy's ability to grow immensely powerful in the USA in the last century is clearly linked to its success in establishing its own medical schools with state charters to grant degrees (chronicled by Coulter[8], the historical analyst).

The same can be said for osteopathy in the USA in the more recent past. To this could be added that the later loss of an independent position from which to challenge orthodoxy from the outside, rather than from the inside, enfeebles the said normal tensions of contrariety emanating from such Biocentric practices whereby the entire sturdy cultural fabric of medicine as a whole has always benefited.

The opportunity

It is very seldom that one has the opportunity to help to develop a cultural element of possibly lasting importance where all the idealistic components can be built in as supportive braces and struts. This may be one of these rare opportunities.

It could be suggested by the collective Biocentric practitionership that the curricula for (a) the medicinal branch and (b) the physical medicine branch of Biocentric Medicine remain as presented previously[1]. Yet, with a view to minimizing mere educational quantification and furthering fuller qualification in tertiary education, ten such supportive aspects are being offered for consideration.

Education manifest for Biocentric Medicine

1. Train Biocentric Medicine lecturers as educators, not as mere experts in content; educational excellence should be rewarded as fully as excellence in biomedical and homoeopharmaceutical research or in clinical practice.

2. Require continuity of education throughout every graduate's life (as a constant learning experience, beginning with admission to the Biocentric Medical school and ending with retirement from active practice) with emphasis away from any passive methods, by rewarding self-directed and independent study – as is more proper for the Empiricist School.

3. Enlarge the range of settings in which internships and other educational exposure is carried through, to include all Biocentric health resources spread throughout the community, not hospitals alone. Generally increase the scope for team-work and joint educational and research opportunities with other Biocentric and health-related

professionals.

4. Allow some flexibility in the content of the Biocentric Medicine curricula to reflect the changing health priorities of the population and the availability of affordable resources.

5. Design the subject content and examination methods in order to achieve both professional competence and the formation of individual as well as social values, not merely the ruminatory memorizing of information.

6. Increase the subject content on active promotion of health and prevention of disease.

7. Ensure that the teaching of research methodology is allied with the admonishment to students that the patient always remains the ultimate and supreme object of a practitioner's quest, next to which scientific investigation must necessarily remain secondary. Similarly the formation of social values (under point 5/) must remain subordinate to the ethical priority of protecting and helping the patient to cure sickness, rather than suggesting that the Biocentric professional is primarily at the disposal of the community.

8. Match admission policies for student enrolment to the population's requirement of Biocentric doctors, and devise and utilize applicant selection methods that can assess positive personal qualities and intuitive faculties.

9. Foster the empiricist skills of questioning, analysis, and an intelligently informed scepticism of authority.

10. Ensure the teaching of both streams of medical history, Rationalist and Empiricist, as well as rudimentary comparative ethnopharmacy and ethnomedicine.

The prospects
The points set out in the Introduction are here briefly readdressed:

Ad 1/ *On an inspired and reflective tertiary education*
The Education Manifest's suggestions (or some of them) could be built into the curricula for Biocentric Medical studies. It is essential that the curricula be as broadly-based as possible, since comparisons and contrasts will immediately be made with that offered by orthodox medical schools. Anything less will be to the Biocentric medical practitioner's permanent disadvantage. The above ten points might as easily become integral parts of any orthodox medical studies, implying that the initiative could be lost for Biocentric Medicine. Whilst this is true, orthodox medical schools have historically only trained students in advanced techniques and facts of medical mechanics. The more genuine educational experience of scientific scepticism by orthodox students is always severely discouraged. For instance, MacEoin has pointed out that textbooks dealing with sociology and politics of orthodox medicine are generally not found in university medical libraries. These will only be found in general libraries[5]. There is resistance to any element philosophically foreign to orthodoxy, and any perceived threat of attendant change, however slight. Orthodoxy's philosophical bedrock is so entrenched that all such educational adaptations will be slow. That means Biocentric Medicine can feel secure in having a significant head-start over orthodoxy for some time to come in this one area.

Ad 2/ *On the EC's perception of Biocentric Medicine* The fears have been shown, *ipso facto*, by this Directive to be largely unfounded. The aim of all EC Governments is to achieve cheap medical treatment, which is what Biocentric medicine offers. This alone will assure it some form of future continuity. The medical ideal that Governments would ike to strive for, as expressed by their embodiment, the World Health Organization (WHO), is that in an educated democracy, citizens should be encouraged to take responsibility for their own health. This means they should be free to pursue methods of self-help (these often turn out to Biocentric methods), or to engage a biomedical practitioner to do this for them. But this has remained an ideal only, because nothing can be done as long as certain old attitudes are maintained by the same politicians who are seemingly awed by mainstream medicine's pervasive technocratic trappings. Yet with the tide of broad public sentiment now turning away from orthodoxy, its attempt to defend its entrenched restrictive privileges is going to be a fascinating exercise in public persuasion. This may already have recently begun. The imponderable element may be the consequence for Biocentric Medicine, should orthodoxy faily in its attempt at public persuasion. Orthodox medicine has powerful advocates in both Houses of Parliament and knows it is fighting a Government which has perhaps taken on just too many opponents at present. The Government, on the other hand, understands how soon a number of aggrieved 'green' minorities add up to an aggrieved majority. Will orthodox medicine, like the political parties, suddenly also don a 'green' mantle?

Ad 3/ *On the question of innate ability versus academic training* Since this alternative will no longer exist in the foreseeable future, this polemic has become irrelevant, except for healers and dowsers.

Ad 4/ *On the need for a set of ethical standards to govern Biocentric health services* See *The Proposal* below.

Ad/5 *On the even diminishing number of options left for self-determination by Biocentric Medicine.* The very substantial growth in popular demand for Biocentric Medical services in recent times has pressed Biocentric Medicine into the public limelight and, therefore, into the area of public concern. The past failure by Biocentric Medicine to regulate itself from within has led to the need for restrictions being imposed from without. The United Kingdom's *Education Reform Act* and this binding EC Directive are the first two of such externally imposed regulatory measures. The next Directive will very probably regulate Biocentric medicines – and without any real input from representatives of the bulk of its prescribers, because no unified representative body for the Biocentric profession will be in a position to speak unambiguously for them. In this area Biocentric medicine dare not rest secure, but must as a matter of utmost urgency, take the initiative and chart its own future course with bold vision, or expect to be regulated and spoken for by outsiders. The obvious fact which has been ignored is that the entire problem needs more than technical solutions. It needs political courage. See *The Proposal* below.

Ad 6/ *On the disunity in the Biocentric leadership* The CCAM and the ICM, in the first half of 1989, have – separately – been engaged in continuing discussions with the Department of Health, the CNAA, the Department of Employment, Training Agency, and the National Council of Vocational Qualifications (NCVQ). WoPACM, on the other hand, has very recently been polling the Biocentric practitionership and the pool of Biocentric therapists for over a year. By this means it has obtained democratic approval for eight *Government Guidelines*, as well as for another eight rudimentary concepts forged into a *Policy Proposals* document. This will be directed, through WoPACM's Parliamentary sub-group, both to the British Government and through them ultimately to the EC. (See *The Proposal* below).

Ad 7/ (i) *On the research programme for Biocentric Medicine* This remains unaffected, except, perhaps, as per 9/ under *The proposal* below.

Ad 7/ (ii) *On the educational programme for Biocentric Medicine* One way of overcoming the multiplicity of curricula would be to establish an Electronic Academy offering such courses through a computerized/audio-visual Biocentric Education Network, with hands-on tutorials at designated centres throughout the country, offered at regular intervals. (See *The Proposal* below).

Ad 8/ (i) & (ii) *On the strong external bipolar influences affecting Biocentric Medicine (from the political arena, as well as from orthodoxy)* Ultimately the world's non-Biocentric medical leadership can be traded back to two organizations: the WHO and the World Medical Association, Inc (WMA). One of these, the WHO, has an established tendency to support non-conventional (traditional) forms of medicine, for politico-economic reasons. It is an international agency run by appointees of world Governments. As a consequence the WHO always ranks political, economic and sociological considerations well above any special-group interests, such as those of orthodox medical associations, which make up the WMA.

The significance of this dichotomy was sharply highlighted in Edinburgh during August 1988, at the time of the World Conference on Medical Education. This was held under the auspices of the World Federation for Medical Education (WFME) and was attended by representatives of the WMA and the WHO (a co-sponsor of the conference). The WHO apparently exerted its influence on the WFME, which pressed for the adoption of *The Edinburgh Declaration* at the conclusion of the Conference. This set out to make the prime aim of future medical education to produce orthodox physicians that would be professionals who would be at the disposal of their community. This was opposed by the WMA, who argued for the practitioner's professional autonomy in serving the best interests and needs of each patient, through the community or not.

The correspondence on this subject between the WMA's Secretary General and the WFME's President has been published in *The World Medical Journal* which comments on this issue (resolved in the WMA's favour) in the following words: "The conclusion of that small story is very simple and clear: there is a deep gap between the medical philosopy defended by the politicians – WHO is a governmental body – and that supported by the medical profession. The former wants to meet the needs defined by the 'Community' and to place the medical doctor at the disposal of the State in order to realize and to facilitate that policy. The latter wants to meet the patients' needs. This is also important, of course, but in environmental circumstances for medical care and the delivery of medical services"[7] (See *The Proposal* below).

Ad 9/ On the threat largely perceived, both by the EC's non-British orthodox medical practitioners, their British counterparts, and paramedics and nurses, many of whom may have 'opted-out' of a restructured Health Service The issue of setting standards to assess whether or not appropriate training would assure professional competence, can only be prosecuted seriously after proper 3 year full-time Biocentric Medical curricula have been brought into existence. These would have to conform to agreed standards previously laid down. Yet this can only be achieved by the authority wielded through a single Board for Biocentric Medicine. The point was made previously in *Complementary Medical Research*[1] that "the stamp of a particular profession and the class of its professionals, that distinguishes them from amateurs, is only forged through education and always maintained by political protection-ism. That is what Biocentric Medicine must aim for now, if it is to flourish as it might". An additional point to be made should be that, as the establishment of the courses has now become obligatory, they ought to be of the highest possible standard to produce a Biocentric practitioner of high calibre (including ex-orthodox paramedics and nursing graduates such as Exeter University intends to cater for), but also to facilitate proper assessment of extraneous professional competence against the standards set through these courses. Without unity in the Biocentric leadership, however, this can never be uniformly achieved and Biocentric Medicine may, seen pessimistically, yet be destined to be ineptly practised by large numbers of inappropriately trained newcomers.

Ad 10/ *On the erosion of Common Law rights that have favoured 'the British way' in the practice of Biocentric Medicine* The absurd but grim paradox appears to be that the less that is done in the British Isles right now con-cerning effective self-regulation in this field of medicine, the more imminent the certainty of precisely this form of erosion occurring through externally imposed, EC-inspired regulation. This is so because, as stated elsewhere[1] through the *Single European Act* of 1986 the British Parliament has effectively abrogated its authority in this area. Those to whom 'the British way' in Biocentric Medicine is dear will urgently want to see their leadership united to enable it to regain the initiative in all Biocentric matters, so as to reinject some of 'the British way' into the relevant sections of whatever the European Parliament may be planning to enact.

Fulder has put the situation in a nutshell: "The freedom under UK common law is an enviable freedom not shared by therapists in other European countries that largely follow the Napoleonic code, in which activaities are generally restricted unless regulations expressly permit them"[8]. There is a profound difference here between British liberality and the restrictiveness permeating the rest of Europe.

In the case of other EC Directives (eg. the *Lingua* Directive) the British Government has vetoed the implementation, saying the British do not like to be told what to do. But in the case of this Directive the Government – for undisclosed reasons – has decided to acquiesce. It has allowed it to become law, which forces the issue. It is reported on good authority, that the osteopaths, the chiropractors and the orthodox practitioners have had representatives and, in two cases, European counsels advising them about the trend of such developments in the EC. As a consequence, the first two were properly prepared with their educational courses and now cannot be excluded. This foresight guarantees them ongoing independence.

Regrettably, this cannot be said for the stewards of the remaining Biocentric disciplines, whose leadership many practitioners and therapists now openly describe as 'navel-gazing'. On the 21st May 1989 a 'Public Interorganization Discussion' was the centrepiece of the Second British Congress of Complementary and Alternative Practitioners (BRICCAP). This was a public summit where the CNAA, ICM, CCAM, the British Chiropractic Association (BCA), EoPACM, the European Further Education Partnership, and MD Associates, faced BRICCAP in open forum under the chairmanship of the editor of the *Journal of Alternative and Complementary Medicine* (JACM) (*see footnote* below†).

---

† Panel Members: Dr Chris Thomson (WoPACM); Dr Alan Hibbert (CNAA); David Ellis (MD Associates); Dr Bill Rust (European Further Education Partnership); Michael Copland-Griffiths (BCA); Ken Shifrin (CCAM); Michael Endacott (ICM). Chairman: Richard Thomas (JACM editor).

Some of the issues raised there made it appear as though there were options open to Biocentric Medicine which by then clearly no longer existed.

This author sees current reality like this: The three year full-time course for Biocentric medical training is now law and must be implemented before 4th January 1991. In the wake of this must come the trappings of some form of registration procedure. This, in turn, implies some supervision of professional practice in accordance with publicly accepted standards of ethics. it also gives rise to the exigence that all Biocentric practices would have to show themselves in some way as compatible with the general systematic body of knowledge. That will reduce the scope of 'intuitive' practices and lead to a likely 'medicalization' of basic Biocentric tenets. That means practitioners and therapists will, sooner rather than later, give up some of their current independence. It also means some of that 'British way' is already gone, having given way to European restrictions.

Accepting that, and acting positively on it now, would quickly place Biocentric medicine in a very strong position in the UK and Eire. Failing to act will simply mean that the stage occupied by Biocentric practitioners and therapists will be taken over by those who consider that they already have an approximate educational equivalent (orthodox practitioners, nurses and paramedics). Those who have laboured till now to take the therapies and practices to where they are at present, will inexorably be sidelined, never to return. (See *The Proposal* below).

The proposal

To provide a solid platform from which to negotiate with Government, the EC and other bodies, consideration is invited to the proposal that WoPACM, after full consultation with both CCAM and ICM, as well as with its own Parliamentary Group, immediately undertake polling all therapists and the full practitionership of Biocentric Medicine, simultaneously along the general lines modelled by the following twelve prototypical questions:

1. Whether or not they would like to have the Government oblige ICM, CCAM, and WoPACM, or a similar organisation, to become a single body, by refusing henceforward to deal with any one of them separately; if answered in the affirmative, then other issues could imediately be canvassed too;

2. Whether such a single representative body should, perhaps, be named the Federal Board for Biocentric Medicine (FBBM); or given some other appropriate name, e.g the Council for Professions Complementary to Medicine as suggested by Brian Inglis;

3. Whether the FBBM, or equivalent, ought to establish – at the earliest opportunity – formal contact with the WHO, which is known to favour strongly the objectives outlined in the *Education Manifest* above and, in any event, would be prepared to regard most of Biocentric Medicine, as practised in the UK and Eire, as the ethnomedicine of the British Isles, which the WHO traditionally supports[9].

4. Whether or not there is approval of each section of the *Education Manifest for Biocentric Medicine* as outlined, or whether, perhaps, there are adverse feelings about (part of) that suggestion;

5. Whether the FBBM, or equivalent, should or should not be empowered to draw up an educational plan in the spirit proposed here and within the restrictions imposed by the EC Directive (it is further suggested that the curricula, which were fully set down previously), be submitted for consideration also to those so polled, as well as the

suggested (electronic computerized/audio-visual) Biocentric Education Network, perhaps as possible alternatives to each other);

6. Whether the FBBM, or equivalent, should be empowered by Government as the Registration Body for the Biocentric Medical profession/therapy of each individual party polled (though it is to remain distinct from the General Medical Council, as well as from such bodies as the General Council and Register of Naturopaths (GCRN), the General Council and Register of Osteopaths (GCRO), the BCA, The British Naturopathic and Osteopathic Association (BNOA), the Organization of Independent Homoeopathic Colleges (OIHC), etc);

7. Whether the FBBM, or equivalent, should draw up a relevant Code of Proper Conduct (which could also lay down strict guidelines on the use of titles and academic epithets), to be made enforceable through the imposition penalties (maximim, to be loss of Registration) after duly constituted disciplinary hearings;

8. Whether or not the courses to be offered here should be advertised in other parts of the EC to attract paying students (from, say, France, where this type of course would not be available) to help to subsidize the costs (this would compete with the existing courses in the FRG – see *The Consequences: 6/* above);

9. Whether the FBBM, or equivalent, should perhaps be endowed in a manner (e.g. empowered to impose 'research levies' on registered practitioners and therapists, and to dispose over such funds) enabling research to be co-ordinated by it, though carried out under the aegis of specialized organizations such as the RCCM and others like it;

10. Whether the FBBM, or equivalent, should be empowered to negotiate with Government, the EC and other-interest groups (e.g. Nursing Council, or bodies representing pharmaceutical interests, etc);

11. Whether the FBBM, or equivalent, should be empowered to prepare draft legislation, after carefully scrutinizing all similar moves toward legislation elsewhere (e.g. in Canada, FRG, USA, South Africa, Mexico, New Zealand, Greece, Australia, PR China, India, USSR, Netherlands, Argentina, PR Bulgaria, Switzerland and the five Scandinavian countries).

12. Whether the FBBM, or equivalent, should supervise and regulate, while actively encouraging, the provision of laboratory testing facilities for Biocentric Medical practitioners, to add an extra dimension to their current observations of external signs, as originally suggested by Lamong[10] and more recently by Fulder[8].

References

1. Gaier HC. Implementation of a resolute educational strategy: essential element to secure the future for non-orthodox medicine. *Comp Med Res* 1989; 3(2): 30–35.
2. Council of Europe. *Legislation and administrative regulations on the use by licensed health service personnel of non-conventional methods of diagnosis and treatment of illness.* Strasbourg: COE, 1984. On completion of a consultative study, the EC's official report concluded that "the persistent and widespread use of non-conventional methods of diagnosis and treatment of disease indicates a public need which is not satisfied by orthodox medicine in our present health care system".

3. Association of Community Health Councils for England and Wales. *The State of Non-Conventional Medicine: the Consumer View.* London: 1988.

4. Thomas R. Editorial comment. *J Alt Comp Med* 1989; 7)4): 5.

5. MacEoin D. Individualism or integration? *J Alt Comp Med* 1989: 7(3): 25.

6. Coulter HL. *Divided Legacy: a History of the Schism in Medical Thought.* 3 vols. Vol 3: *Science and Ethics in American Medicine 1800–1914.* Washington: Wehawken Book Co, 1973, p304.

7. World Medical Journal. Medical education: WFME in Edinburgh. *World Med J* 1988; 35(6): 90–93.

8. Fulder S. *The Handbook of Complementary Medicine.* 2nd ed. Oxford: OUP, 1988, p65.

9. World Health Organization. *The Promotion of Traditional Medicine.* Geneva: WHO, 1978. (Technical Report series no. 622).

10. Lamont K. The value of blood tests in diagnosis. *J Res Soc Nat Therap* 1975; July.

CHAPTER 2

Complementary medicine in Europe: some natural perspectives

David Aldridge

Summary

The delivery of health care in Europe occurs in a context of dynamic change which is being influenced by consumer demands and imminent European Community legislation. There are no common sets of data to compare between the differing countries. Each country has its own dynamic tradition of health care. Complementary medicine appears to be used by particular sub-cultures. We have little understanding of how much of their disposable income people are willing to allocate to their health care needs, nor how they decide what those particular health care needs are. For complementary practices to be validated they will need to provide some form of scientific evidence which is currently lacking. Active collaboration between groups and national organisations may provide comparative data sets.

Introduction

Throughout Europe there is a growing awareness of complementary medical approaches. Some of the initiatives for this awareness have come from the lay consumers of health care despite the overall monopoly of Western scientific medicine[1,2,3].

If complementary medicine is to be used as a complement within the wide context of health care then there needs to be some assessment of the relative costs compared with orthodox medicine, the extent to which complementary medical approaches can be practised in a pluralistic health care culture and a broad understanding of health care needs in the future. These needs will be determined by the producers (medical personnel), the providers (insurance companies and Government departments) and the consumers (patients)[1].

Any assessment of costs which leads to policy decisions will depend upon accurate research data.

In 1989 there has been an initiative within the EEC to consider the impact of complementary medicine on health care delivery. Within the framework of the Fourth Medical and Health Research Programme, adopted by the Council of the Ministers of the European Communities to stimulate European collaboration in medical and health research, there have been two meetings. The first was an expert meeting held in Brussels in February 1989. From this expert meeting several participants from European states were invited to a workshop to discuss a European concerted action research programme.

The workshop was organized to develop a formal research proposal for concerted action which would consider the integration of complementary medicine within health care delivery. The main aim of the work was to seek agreement on the appropriate research methodology for European research into the integration of complementary medicine within health care delivery. To achieve this aim it was necessary to gather some idea of the extent of the practice of complementary medicine throughout Europe[4,6,7–10].

In the following section of this book the reader will find detailed papers from seven social scientists working in the field of complementary medicine and health care delivery.

Guy Sermeus[8] is project officer with the Belgian

Consumer's Association and responsible for social science research projects and has a great deal of experience concerning survey research methods.

Niels Rasmussen[7] and Janine Morgall are sociologists working at the Danish Institute for Epidemiology.

Kate Thomas is a social scientist in the Department of Community Medicine at the University of Sheffield. It was her initiative and energy which promoted this research collaboration.

Françoise Bouchayer[5] is also a social scientist. She works at the Mission Recherche Experimentation with the Ministry of Social Affairs and Employment.

Tuuala Vaskilampi[9] is Acting Professor of Social Studies at the University of Jyväsklä in Finland and has extensive knowledge of both complementary medicine and traditional practices.

Joost Visser[10] works within the context of orthodox medicine at the Netherlands Institute of Primary Health Care. This organisation is currently co-operating with the World Health Organisation to investigate methods of delivering primary health care.

It will be apparent to the reader that the German article leans heavily on philosophy and has no objective data as do the other papers. The problem is that in Germany, although there are statistics gathered from various organisations, these statistics have not yet been collated within one report. Such a collation is currently being undertaken for the German government.

Discussion

There are some common themes to these various initatives, although there are no homogenous sets of statistics common to all participating countries in the European community. Overall, the state of complementary medicine is rather dynamic, occurring as it does at a time of social change. There are soon to be imposed legislative changes regulating the practice. As Vaskilampi points out in her article, policy making inevitably restricts 'alternatives' which are free from restraint and outside of the system. Some ethnic practices flourish precisely because they are un-regulated[11]. The attainment of the status of complementarity will be for the powerful and organised few. Alternatives, however, will remain. Should certain practitioners be forced underground through hasty and ill founded legislation, then the public will be prey to quackery and criminality. Tolerance of alternatives is an indicator of our cultural maturity. Therapeutic repression will only bring about the problems which the 'quack' hunters fear.

Social aspects

It might appear from a cursory examination of the statistics that it is the middle-aged, worried, well woman who is the prime user of complementary medicine. Complementary medicines do not appear to be used so much by those under eighteen years and those over 60 years of age. The lack of use by those under eighteen may be linked to there being fewer chronic health problems in this group and to family perceptions of appropriate health care.

There is only a little evidence so far about the motivation of patients to use complementary medicines. It could well be that clear groups of users emerge from a carefully administered population survey.

This lack of clarity about why people seek and use alternatives raises an important issue for research into health care delivery. We have yet really to understand the relevance of differing health care systems for particular cultural settings. This comparative understanding of symbolic reality is essential for health care delivery[11]. The activity of healing is a complex process where disease causation, disease classification and the healing act are given some form of coherence according to the appropriate medical ideologies and relevant language[13]. Health care cannot be restricted to one single symbolic medical reality for Europe.

In Finland, for example, acupuncture is incorporated within orthodox or 'school' medicine and is thereby not complementary. It would be interesting to see how the practice of acupuncture, and the symbolic meanings associated with such practice, changes within a modern context of medical orthodoxy compared with a modern context of complementary medicine and a context of traditional practice.

Health economics

Any research into the use of complementary medicines will need to consider the role of disposable income and health care consumption. If a plurality of health care approaches is offered, then it will be necessary to see if there are any substitution effects of one medical approach for another. This will have implications for cost as complementary medicines are often considered to be less expensive than orthodox medicine. At the moment some of the costs of complementary practice are hidden in that general practitioners in some countries practice complementary medicine[1,8,10], but these costs are masked by the general statutory provision of non-specific reimbursement.

A further hidden cost, which is difficult to assess, is the use of self-treatment. Many people, before they see a practitioner, complementary or otherwise, attempt to solve their problem using medicine bought over the counter. It appears that there is a growing use of herbal products to satisfy this demand. Indeed the orthodox/complementary debate may be a distortion of what is really a debate about the relationship between self/family/community care and primary care. Any system which is dependent upon organised consultation becomes expensive. Therefore, initiatives which promote self care and prevention are potentially cheaper. However, such proposals remove some of the monopolist tendencies of health care organisations, be they orthodox or complementary.

In any system of health care it will be necessary to provide quality of care criteria so that patients as consumers can ascertain their own satisfaction; practitioners as producers can meet the demands of providers and patients; and insurers as providers can ensure a recognised standard of provision. Such quality of care criteria are linked to the approved status of practitioners and the reimbursement policies of insurance schemes. There need to be clear guidelines for policy. These should be readily available from the experiences of other EEC member states.

Scientific validation

In general there has been little scientific validation of the effects of these complementary medicines. This has been compounded by two factors: an unwillingness on behalf of the complementary therapists to submit their work for validation[12]; and a lack of research funding, including the political will to provide that research funding, by Governmental bodies[2].

The difficulties of research in the field of complementary medicine are that:

a) the appropriate and necessary research methods have not been developed,

b) orthodox scientific approaches are often insensitive to the needs of some complementary practitioners,

c) there is no broad base of academic research in complementary medicine (although there are some promising initiatives),

d) and that complementary practitioners, not trained in a university environment, have no research expertise.

The difficulties of research into the efficacy of complementary medicine, and the aforementioned quality of care criteria, are based on the notion of medicine as a symbolic reality. With the increased technicalization of modern medicine efficacy and quality of life are separated from practice. While we have ever refined measures of morbidity, mortality and clinical outcome from an orthodox perspective, we have little knowledge of personal, familial and social standards of efficacy and quality according to other cultural criteria. There is then a need for:

1. Research methods appropriate for complementary medicine and sensitive to the practice of that medicine.
2. A co-ordinated policy of research funding.
3. Research consultancy, advice and training for complementary therapists.
4. Co-operative projects between orthodox medical researchers and complementary practitioners.
5. Co-operation between EEC member states for the comparison of data and sharing of expertise. To meet these above needs it would be useful to identify a national central agency which could co-ordinate and develop activities within a member state and foster co-operation between other states. The satisfaction of these needs can also be achieved in the context of long term research planning, co-operation in developing research strategies and international symposia.

Education
It is quite clear that the majority of recognised reimbursed complementary practice is carried out by those with university medical training, and this precedent may be applied to British legislation in any interpretation of European directives. A mandatory directive from the European Community (January 1989) suggests governmentally recognised tertiary education of three years duration for complementary health practitioners. This will

establish a European standard which can also be interpreted locally. Such a system will require practitioners moving from one country to another to learn the local medical and legal precedents.

Germany has a tradition of accreditation and state licensing of practitioners. Orthodox medical practitioners who wish to apply methods of *Heilpraktik* must undergo further training at accredited colleges. (Such qualifications already have some validity within the EC). However, the notion of *Heilpraktiker* is once more being questioned within Germany, reinforcing the notion that in the face of European legislation and internal pressure therapeutic freedom must be continually defended. In the Netherlands governmental initiatives have taken steps to ascertain what is necessary for policy making decisions regarding complementary medicines. While neither of these endeavours may be perfect, it may be to our advantage to learn what they have to offer.

With the development of graduate and postgraduate courses within British universities there can surely be opportunities for our differing institutions to offer co-operative training schemes and research placements. Within the EEC budget there is money available for groups from varying countries to collaborate in shared curricula, and for institutions to learn to co-operate.

References
1. Aldridge D. The delivery of health care alternatives in Europe. *J Roy Soc Med* 1990; 83: 179–182.
2. Fulder S. *The Handbook of Complementary Medicine.* 2nd edition. London: Coronet, 1988.
3. Leibrich J, Hickling J, Pitt G. *In Search of Well Being: Exploratory Research into Complementary Therapies.*

Wellington, New Zealand: Health Services Research and Development Unit, 1987.

4. Bossy J. Legal practice of acupuncture in France. Background paper to the European workshop *The Impact of Non-orthodox Medicine on Health Care Expenditure. Utrecht, the Netherlands, 5–7th June 1989.*

5. Bouchayer F. A general approach to the French situation. Background paper to the European workshop *The Impact of Non-orthodox Medicine on Health Care Expenditure. Utrecht, the Netherlands, 5–7th June 1989.*

6. Lacey L. Alternative medicine in Ireland. Report on the European workshop *The Impact of Non-orthodox Medicine on Health Care Expenditure. Utrecht, the Netherlands, 5–7th June 1989.*

7. Rasmussen N. Use of alternative health care in the Danish adult population. Background paper to the European workshop *The Impact of Non-orthodox Medicine on Health Care Expenditure. Utrecht, the Netherlands, 5–7th June 1989.*

8. Sermeus G. Alternative health care in Belgium: an explanation of various social aspects. Background paper to the European workshop *The Impact of Non-orthodox Medicine on Health Care Expenditure. Utrecht, the Netherlands, 5–7th June 1989.*

9. Vaskilampi T. Alternative medicine in Finland. Background paper to the European workshop *The Impact of Non-orthodox Medicine on Health Care Expenditure. Utrecht, the Netherlands, 5–7th June 1989.*

10. Visser J. Alternative medicine in the Netherlands. Background paper to the European workshop *The Impact of Non-orthodox Medicine on Health Care Expenditure. Utrecht, the Netherlands, 5–7th June 1989.*

11. Kleinman A. Indigenous systems of healing: questions for professional, popular and folk care. In *Alternative Medicines: Popular and Policy Perspectives*, edited by JW Salmon, pp138–164. London: Tavistock Publications, 1984.

12. Watt J. *ed. Talking Health: Conventional and Complementary Approaches.* London: Royal Society of Medicine, 1988.

13. Kleinman A. Medicine's symbolic reality. *Inquiry,* 1973, 16: 206–213.

CHAPTER 3

Alternative medicines: a general approach to the French situation

Françoise Bouchayer

Summary

In France there has been a steady increase in the use of alternative medicines since 1970. Alternative medicines are a mixed group of varying disciplines. While the validity of homoeopathy and acupuncture is being debated by the Academy of Science, prescriptions and consultations to which they give rise are reimbursed by Social Security payments. No alternative medical discipline is taught at a national level.

In a survey of 1000 people in 1985, 49% of the people questioned had already used alternative medicine. Homoeopathy is most widely used (32%) followed by acupuncture (21%).

As much as 7% of health care expenditure in France is linked to alternative medicine. Some alternative health care costs are hidden within general health reimbursements. The majority of complementary mutual insurance schemes do not reimburse alternative medicine. Although some private insurance schemes have reimbursement rates, they are linked to approved practitioners.

Introduction

In France, since around the middle of the 1970s, alternative medicines have been the subject of increasing social success. The number of practitioners, doctors and non-doctors, as well as the number of users of these medicines have increased substantially. In parallel, the cultural and media-related products devoted to these questions have grown strongly, in particular aimed at the general public; books, magazines, exhibitions, radio or television programmes, initiation courses etc. The phenomenon is therefore moving well beyond the strict bounds of the care distribution system and it is rightly often qualified as a 'social phenomenon'.

As far as public authorities are concerned, no really new legislative order has been made in this area over the last few years. However, between 1982 and 1986, the government requested the setting up of two committees. The first was entrusted to Dr Niboyet (acupuncture doctor) and led to a document entitled *Rapport sur certaines techniques de soins ne faisant pas l'objet d'un enseignement organisé au national* (Report about certain care techniques not forming the subject of nationally organized teachings). This report refers to a highly reserved standpoint concerning theoretical references and therapeutic values of most alternative medicines. However, it did introduce certain recommendations made in favour of the teaching of homoeopathy, acupuncture and manual medicine in medical faculties.

The second committee, led by a thinking group consisting of doctors, researchers and representatives of user associations led to the publication of a report *Les médecines différentes, un défi?* (The different medicines, a challenge?)[2]. It outlined standpoints – sometimes divergent – of the different parties confronting one another with respect to a desirable policy in the terms of the qualification and training of practitioners and the evaluation of the therapeutic efficiency of different medicines. This report also underscored the importance of social diffusion obtained by non-orthodox medicines. Because of the governmental change which took place during 1986 (and the departure of Mme Georgina Dufoix, Minister of Social Affairs and Employment), this consultation did not lead to any new measures being made.

As far as research into alternative medicines is concerned, two major areas should be considered: that of bio-medical and clinical research, and that of the sciences of man and of society. The information given in the text relative to the research accomplished already, or under-way, in France, concerns only the social sciences. In this area of research, few works have so far been devoted to different medicines.

Defining alternative medicine

Several terms are used to qualify the care methods in France which do not fall within the sphere of conventional medicine: 'natural', 'parallel', 'alternative', 'different', 'non-official', 'heterodox', 'non-proven'. 'gentle' therapies, etc. While the general public often talks about 'médicines douces' (gentle medicines), the term 'different medicines' is preferred for official use.

For the Ministry of Health and the representatives of the medical profession, one of the main points which is common to the different alternative medicines is the fact that they are not taught at a national echelon in medical faculties. Another parameter which is put forward to attempt to define these medicines is that of their heterodox character concerning doctrinal and epistemological bases of official bio-medicine. For example, we might refer to the infinitesimal notion and the law of similiture in homoeopathy, the concept of energy and references to Taoism for acupuncture, and the principle of 'primary breathing movements' for functional osteopathy. However, other medicines which are also qualified as alternatives do not appear to be far removed, from the doctrinal standpoint, from official medicine; at this point, we might mention phytotherapy or structural osteopathy.

Researchers in social sciences who dealt with such questions took this institutional and epistemological data into consideration, while adding to it a historical viewpopint and principles of definition based on the examination of the current usage of such medicines as an extension of their social diversity, 'innovations', and types of practitioners implementing these care modes (doctors and/or non-doctors)[3,4].

In the perspective of research development into alternative medicines, attempts at definition must take account of social processes without exclusively attempting to establish typologies which more often than not do not prove to be very satisfactory. Among such social processes we might mention:

1) Influences which goven the permanent 'invention' of new labels, if not new therapies. Indeed, there is an almost constant multiplication of alternative care techniques (meso-kinergy, osteodynamics, meso-energy, etc). As far as most of them are concerned, these new therapies are derivatives or associations of derivatives of 'mother disciplines' such as acupuncture, bio-energy, manual medicine. Some are economic, professional, psychological and cultural logics which explain this phenomena of disparity. Who are the people who promote such therapies?

2) The breakdowns between the area of different medicines and the different adjacent sectors such as regular medicine, but also the entire field of psycho-bodily therapies; that of popular medicines (traditional healing practices); the field of the sacred and of religious beliefs (healing by faith and prayer); and finally, and the 'para-scientific' sphere (or of esoteric beliefs and practices) such as astrology, seerism, phenomena of communication at a distance.

The borders between what forms the field of different

others are far less well equipped. It should be
ed that in particular, as far as osteopathy and
ncture are concerned, some practitioners declare
ey were trained on the 'compagnonage' basis (ie. by
g with a qualified and experienced practitioner).
ype of apprenticeship may or may not be a
ment to more 'scholarly' training[6].

umber of schools and training courses in alterna-
dicines has increased substantially over the last 15
so. Alongside the 'benchmark' schools which
heir letters of legitimacy in the field of different
s (even if the diplomas they issue are not officially
d), many more or less 'serious' training centres
founded.

enerally, the field of different medicines in France
structured and institutionalised. One important
e emphasised is that the major therapeutic and
disciplines (acupuncture, homoeopathy, phy-
osteopathy) do not form consistent wholes.
h of these medicines there are doctrinal splits
nd the institutional splits that exist (among the
practitioners, training schools, knowledgeable
c).

e, much research has been devoted to practi-
ifferent medicines on the basis of original data
surveys by questionnaires or by conversations).
forms part of what we might well call the
the health professions; a study of the
and social trajectories, positioning on the care
ice of practising conventional or fee-free
trinal and therapeutic orientations, relations
onal groups (unions, knowledgeable com-
methods of legitimisation through the acquisi-
ledge, by 'donation', by reference to major
ions, etc.

interesting area of research consists of

medicines and what belongs to other social practice areas
must be placed somewhere, but where?

The legal framework in which alternative medicine is situated

When applied to the practice of alternative medicines, the
legislative bases of the health system in France generate a
series of ambiguities and paradoxes. They are extensively
due to the fact that official recognition of different
medicines is primarily part of an action of legitimation (or
of non-legitimation) by such and such an authority, and in
reality has little to do with actually being entered into the
laws applying to the different categories of players and of
institutions concerned. Thus, while homoeopathy, and to a
lesser extent acupuncture, are disciplines whose validity is
still being contested by the Academy of Medicine,
prescriptions or medical consultations to which they give
rise are codified and reimbursed by the Social Security and
have been for several years and are thus blessed by their
backing.

Similarly, no alternative therapy (including the most
widespread acupuncture; homoeopathy, phytotherapy,
osteopathy), is the subject of teaching at a national level.
Except for the DUMENAT (Diplôme Universitaire de
Médicines Naturelles), issued by a university in the Paris
area (Bobigny), there are no officially recognised qualifications in the field. Indeed, certificates or diplomas for
homoeopathy or acupuncture, issued by certain medical
faculties, are not considered as official national diplomas.
Obviously, the same applies to diplomas issued by a great
many private schools. However, any doctor can declare
himself to be a homoeopath or an acupuncturist, regardless
of any additional training he may or may not have
followed.

More generally, in France there is a two-fold movement
as far as the legitimation of the practice of alternative

medicine is concerned, at doctors' level. First, there is a loosening up, or even an opening up, by most of the official authorities (medical professional organisations, faculties of medicine, Ministry of Health, etc) with respect to these doctors. Second, there is greater vigilance, in particular among the medical profession, regarding the conditions under which these medicines are applied and the struggle against medical charlatans (even within the medical profession), regarding prescriptions for natural therapies in the case of serious illness for instance. This vigilance is becoming apparent through the increased number of appearances of doctors before disciplinary boards. From the legislative standpoint, the keystone is the freedom that the doctor is legally entitled to in prescribing therapy that he considers appropriate to the case being dealt with.

However, alternative medicine in France is practised not only by doctors. The main legal problem that arises is due to the fact that doctors have a monopoly for exercising medicine (drawing up diagnosis and decisions regarding therapeutic behaviour). However, many non-doctors, in particular kinesiotherapists, have been trained in non-orthodox therapies and claim the right to practise acupuncture, osteopathy and other alternative therapeutic disciplines. The fact that there is no official regulation concerning acupuncturists, osteopaths, naturopaths etc. forms a legal loophole giving a great deal of the European market dispositions which should come into effect in 1992. For their part, doctors – acupuncturists and osteopaths in particular – are very actively organising matters to deal with such claims and to ensure a monopoly for the distribution of alternative care.

Number and characterists of therapists

Because there is no regulation concerning alternative medical 'specialities', the number of practitioners cannot be evaluated with any accuracy. This is particularly so in

---

the case of non-doctor therapists.

Several estimates agree on the r doctors as approximately 10,000 homoeopathic doctors is betwee number of osteopaths estimated a Among them, is there any reaso doctors who make exclusive therapies and those who imple nally?

According to a survey in 19 range of 200 general practiti investigated declared that th alternative methods (in France general practitioners working these 46%, 5.4% used them often, 72.8% used them oc Approximately one GP in regularly by alternative th similar results.

Doctors using unortho greater part general practit pediatricians (even if thi toward homoeopathy an coming interested in ac Sophrology appears to dentists and midwives.

The number of kine apies can be estimated 25,700 kinesiotherapis

It is thought that th no official diploma as there are many nat evaluate; it must be

The type and le doctors or non-do (perhaps the great

while
obser
acupu
that th
workir
This t
comple
The
tive me
years o
obtain t
medicine
recognise
have bee
More
is strongl
point to
heterodox
totherapy,
Within ea
which ext
unions of
societies, e
In Franc
tioners of
collections
This work
sociology o
professional
market (ch
systems), do
with profess
panies, etc),
tion of know
cultural tradit
One very

analysing for a particular country at a particular time; within a given therapy the links and the connections between the regulations in force on the one hand, and on the doctrinal privileged therapeutic orientations on the other, for categories of practitioners (doctors or non-doctors). On this point, the case of osteopathy might reveal much information.

Frequency of use and patients' characteristics

The main source of quantitative information relative to users of alternative medicines is a survey carried out in 1985 among a representative sample of 1000 people[7]. Forty-nine per cent of the people questioned had already used alternative medicine "if only just once". (This figure was 46% the previous year.) Unfortunately, the formulation of the question did not enable us to evaluate the recent or the previous type of treatment, or the frequency employed.

Again, according to this survey, the alternative medicine most widely used is homoeopathy (32%), followed by acupuncture (21%), phytotherapy (12%), chiropractic (4%) and osteopathy (3%).

Recourse to alternative medicine appears to be particularly frequent among executives and higher intellectual professions (68%), average executives and intermediate professions (60%), artisans, traders, company managers (57%), and other employees (52%). Farmers (40%) appear to be relatively less frequent users of different medicines.

44% of men and 53% of women have had recourse to these medicines. The highest percentages are to be found in the 35–45 years age group (59%), followed by the 50–64 years (50%), then the 25–34 years (45%). Other surveys reveal similar results, in particular concerning the socio-professional distribution of the users.

An extensive survey into the living conditions carried out in 1987 by INSEE (Institut National de la Statistique et des Etudes Economiques) among 13,000 people, brought together a complete series of questions concerning health. One of them had to give new statistics regarding the use of alternative medicine (this survey is currently under review).

Beyond a few soundings very little work has been devoted in France to users of alternative medicines. In any forthcoming research, two points should be emphasised:

1) The users of alternative medicines are not a separate category of health care consumers. It is the pattern of consumption between recourse to orthodox medicine and alternative medicine which is interesting to study. The notion of a therapeutic career, ie. a succession of varying resources as used by the same patient over a particular time period, can be a fruitful subject for studying health care usage.

2) Social, cultural and psychological determinacies which govern the orientation of users toward alternative medicines are extremely diversified. Some users are mainly in quest of efficient and non-iatrogenous therapies, while others are 'human' practitioners (slow medicine, 'listening' medicine etc). Others yet again are strongly attracted and interested in the universe of philosophies and beliefs about Man, his position in the universe, the meaning of existence etc, and choose a therapy which fits in with this philosophy[8].

Patient satisfaction

The aforementioned survey[5] included a question regarding the evaluation of alternative medicine efficiency according to the experience of the integrated users themselves. Seventy per cent estimate that these therapies are efficient for minor ailments (such as flu, colds, general fatigue, headaches), 65% for chronic symptoms (sleeplessness, rheumatism, digestive problems, allergies), 9% for serious ailments (cancer, cardiac problems etc). Conversely, only 11% consider that these therapies are not very or are not at all efficient for minor ailments, 15% for chronic symptoms, 38% for serious illnesses. For each of these three problem categories, respectively 19%, 20% and 53% of alternative medicine users have nothing to report.

Forty-nine per cent of users have consulted doctors for minor ailments, 54% for chronic symptoms, 3% for serious illnesses, and 17% for preventive medicine and a healthy lifestyle.

It might be possible to carry out, as part of research into human and social sciences, an approach towards the notion of the efficiency and results of therapeutic interventions, which have now broken free of the conventional biomedical approaches. What status should be given to the notion of patient satisfaction, to the evaluation of the effects of care? How can this dimension be taken into account at a methodological level?

Economic implementations: financial aspects and reimbursement

Some writers consider that between 3.5% and 7% of the total health expenditure in France is spent on alternative medicine, excluding the alternative care provided within a hospital framework. On this point, we might emphasise an increase in the number of homoeopathy and acupuncture consultations made in a hospital environment over the last 10 years or so.

We have already mentioned the fact that acupuncture sessions and homoeopathic prescriptions are reimbursed by the Social Security provided the doctor who issues them is an agreed doctor. In addition, even if they are not the subject of specific codification, medical phythotherapy consultations, consultations for different therapies, or alternative technical sessions by an approved kinesiotherapist, are reimbursed by the Social Security. More often than not, the Social Security is 'unaware' of the alternative or other nature of the service provided. Conversely, costs linked with the purchase of phytotherapy products are not recognised in any way.

Currently there is no way of evaluating the respective proportion of the shared costs assumed by the users and Social Security with regard to alternative pharmaceuticals and alternative health care.

We can be sure that the user's share of the cost of alternative care is substantially more than his share of the cost of regular care. Indeed, the proportion of acupuncturists, homoeopathic and osteopathic doctors who have chosen the free fees area is substantially higher than that of practitioners of conventional specialities. Since 1982, doctors working on a freelance basis have had the pssibility, while remaining within the conventions established between the Medical Unions and the Social Security, to choose between 'sector I' of this convention (in which case, they agree to abide by conventional prices) or 'sector II'. In the latter case, the doctor freely establishes the amount of his fees; the patient, on the other hand, is paid only on the basis of the conventional price. In addition, homoeopaths or acupuncturists more frequently chose that their· colleagues no longer agreed at all; consultation fees are then fully at the expense of the patient.

The annual fees for acupuncture and homeopathy are lower than in general practice for two reasons; the practitioners themselves are often young professionals (still building up their reputation), and the consultation time for acupuncture and homoeopathy is longer than that in general practice.

Among kinesiotherapists, there is no free fee area. Because of the difficulty of compatibility between the operations conducted by an alternative kinesiotherapist –

Table 1

1988	Sector 1	Free fees	Non-agreed
homoeopathic doctors	12.9%	81.5%	4.5%
acupuncture doctors	24.3%	72.5%	2.8%
general practitioner doctors	84.3%	14.4%	0.4%
specialist doctors	62.0%	27.2%	0.3%

Conversely, the amount of prescriptions issued in the homoeopathic medical field is substantially less than in the regular medicine field and is almost nil for acupuncture.

From these statistics drawn up by the Social Security among doctors practicing homoeopathy and acupuncture, the average overall amount of the annual fees received appears to be less than that of regular general practitioners (in 1988) –

- homoeopathic doctors: 393,096 FF
- acupuncture doctors: 414,728 FF
- general practitioners: 481,731 FF
- specialist doctors: 804,013 FF

The amount of consultation fees are, respectively, in 1988 and for sectors I's doctors:

- general practitioners: 85 FF
- specialist practitioners: 125 FF
- acupuncture practitioners: 72 FF

Free fees asked by sector II's homoeopathic and acupuncture doctors generally varied between 150 FF and 250 FF.

osteopathy for instance – which demands much time, and the 'conventional' price rates established for the profession, an increasing number of kinesiotherapists are surveying their patients on a 'non-conventionalised' basis or on a totally 'de-conventionalised' basis. The same applies for kinesiotherapists who practise acupuncture. In these cases, costs are fully born by the user.

The great majority of complementary mutual insurance schemes do not ensure complementary reimbursement of care fees when the practitioner is 'approved', even more so within the limits of the price lists in sector I. Several private insurance schemes propose more interesting complementary reimbursement rates for medical fees in sector II (but no reimbursement for non-agreed (*non conventionnes*) practitioner fees.

More research is needed on the financial aspects of supply and consumption of alternative medicine, and its position within France's health economy.

Conclusion

In the perspective of comparative European research relating to alternative medicines, we would suggest the following:

1) Encourage people to develop work based on rigorous empirical data. Indeed, it would appear that many recent publications correspond more to general thinking about alternative medicines and their social usages than to real and original research work. This refers directly back to the question of appropriate methodologies which must be quantitative and qualitative, and allow comparative approaches etc. .

2) Produce relevant guidelines showing the level of integration of alternative medicines in the Health Systems of individual countries, and to follow their developments. Is there not a trend toward the redevelopment of integration between alternative medicines on the one hand and conventional medicines on the other? Indeed, will not gradual recognition of the part of different alternative medicines go hand in hand with the radicalisation of an entire sector of social practices relative to these same medicines?

In spite of its apparent homogeneity, the current success of alternative medicines is due to very diverse influences. They therefore fall within social movements which are inherent to the future of medicine and health, but also to the aspirations and social-cultural evolutions of a more general nature. These different influences must be considered in perspective for all of the points dealt with in this text.

In terms of research questions, we might consider carrying out comparative analysis between the different European countries on questions such as:

– offsets between legislations in the health area and existing practices,

– the complex non-monolithic character of this legislation and the ambiguities or paradoxes resulting from it,

– the modifications, adaptations and regulation retained in an attempt to integrate – or to combat – the development of certain practices and of certain practitioners.

References
1. Niboyet E H. *Rapport sur certaines Techniques de Soin ne faisant pas L'Objet d'un Enseignement organisé au Niveau National.* Maisonneuve, 1984.
2. *Les Medicines Differentes, un Defi? Rapport au Ministère des Affaires Sociales et de la Solidarité Nationale et au Sécretaire d'Etat Chargé de la Santé. Paris: Documentation Française, 1988.*
3. Barel Y, Butel A M. *Le Medicines Paralleles quelques Lignes de Force MIRE.* Paris: Documentation Française, 1988.

4. Bouchayer F, La nebuleuse des autres medicines: essai de cartographic. *Etudes* 1986; Oct: 317–330.

5. *Impact Medicin* 1987; (217) 14–20 March.

6. Bouchayer F. Médicines différentes, parcours de généralistes. *Prospective et Santé* 1985; 34 (Summer): 43–50.

7. *Médicines Douces* 1985; (47) Dec.

8. Bouchayer F. Les usagers des médicines alternatives: itineraires therapeutiques, culturels, existentiels. *Revue Francaise des Affaires Sociales* 1986; May (no. hors-serie): 105–115.

CHAPTER 4

Alternative health care in Belgium: an explanation of various social aspects

Guy Sermeus

Summary

To practice any form of medicine in Belgium it is necessary to be enrolled with the Belgian General Medical Council. Recognised doctors have clinical and diagnostic freedom to carry out whatever treatments they see fit. Those who choose to practice complementary medicine may find themselves in conflict with their professional organisation which requires them to treat patients "taking all reasonable care given the current state of scientific knowledge".

General practitioners offer most of the available homoeopathy and acupuncture. Physiotherapists provide most of the osteopathy.

Alternative health care is not reimbursed by the social security system although there is evidence that patients would like the cost of alternative health care to be reimbursed. About one in four Belgians consult a complementary practitioner, perhaps the highest use of alternative health care in Europe.

Legal measures regarding alternative health care in Belgium.

The practice of medicine in Belgium must be considered within the framework of an absolute monopoly for doctors. This situation is the result of history, and is to a large extent based on a law dating from before the foundation of Belgium, that of 12 March 1818, "regarding the regulation of the exercise of the various tasks of the healing arts" and the Statutory Instrument of 31 May 1818, "concerning a regulation regarding medical research and care"[1].

The intention was to bring about standardisation within the maze of different job areas and persons practising medicine. The "representatives of the Provincial Medical Commissions", who themselves were "practitioners in one of the medical fields" were entrusted by article 4c of the Law of 1818 with the responsibility of "supervision of the good and proper performance of the practise of medical science and of all having to do with the health of the population in general"[2].

Medical schools were given the power to grant degrees as doctors in medicine, surgery and obstetrics (MB BCh), from 1876 onwards[3]. The second level schools were abolished and the secondary grades – surgeon, officer of health – were seldom awarded by the provincial medical commissions. The Law on Higher Education of 15 July 1849 recognised the degree of 'doctor of medicine, surgery and obstetrics' as the sole legal degree qualification. Those qualifications recognised by previous legislation, but now no longer valid, were protected by transitional provisions. It was not until the beginning of the 20th century that all doctors held the same sole valid degree of 'doctor of medicine, surgery and obstetrics' and these were then drawn together in one professional body.

The Belgian GMC was set up under the Law of 25 July 1938[4]. Because of the war this body could not begin to function until 1947[5]. Membership of the Belgian GMC is compulsory in order to be able to practice medicine. Membership is restricted to persons in possession of a degree as 'doctor of medicine, surgery and obstetrics'.

From the measures discussed above it can be seen that in Belgium there is legally speaking no room for free practice of medicine – whatever definition is given of this practice – by persons who are not enrolled with the Belgian GMC as doctors. Persons practising alternative medical or even allopathic medicine under such conditions commit a criminal offence.

On the other hand, it is the case that doctors of 'medicine, surgery and obstetrics' enjoy clinical and diagnostic freedom. They can thus use any methods or techniques which can justifiably contribute to making a diagnosis or carrying out a treatment. So called alternative treatments fall within the bounds of this clinical and diagnostic freedom and may be used perfectly legally. However, the 'Code of Medical Ethics', while recognising this clinical and diagnostic freedom, clearly indicates the limited nature of this freedom[6]. Thus it is assumed that when a doctor agrees to treat a patient, he must do so taking all reasonable care given the current state of scientific knowledge.

Complementary medicine is not taught in Belgian medical schools, at least not as part of the official syllabus for a 'doctor of medicine, surgery and obstetrics'. The reason for this is that they are seen by the Belgian Royal College of Physicians as being scientifically insufficiently proven or unprovable. Although this occurs less and less frequently, it is possible that a fully qualified doctor could be called before the Belgian GMC for practising the techniques of alternative therapy. What happens more frequently is that the Belgian GMC will prosecute non-doctors for practising alternative therapies. The reason for the prosecution is thus not 'using alternative medicine' but 'illegal practice of medicine'.

The extent of alternative health care in Belgium
There is a relatively small number of studies on the subject of alternative health care and, in addition, the attention of researchers has turned to this area only fairly recently.

Until 1983 there were in fact no numerical research studies available to give any systematic quantitative data regarding alternative health care.

The first series of estimates was based on extrapolations from various partial or specific research observations which give national percentage figures based on what frequently are incompletely thought out hypotheses. In 1981 J Van Hecke estimated that 10%–12% of the Belgian population made use of AHC (Alternative Health Care) for the purpose of attempting to solve various health problems[7]. In 1982 he repeats these figures[8]. In 1984 Guy Sermeus suggested a significantly higher usage figure of between 18% and 28% This refers to persons of 18 years of age and older who have ever made use of any form of AHC carried out by a practitioner. This author added that the greater part of this usage of alternative medicine within this period probably occurred within a limited period of time, specifically during the last 2–3 years[9].

In 1984, at the initiative of the Ministry for the Flemish Community, Department of Health Administration, a representative study was carried out with the intention of quantifying the extent of use of AHC[10]. The survey was carried out by the IIVO (Universitaire Instituut voor Voorming en Ontwikkeling) which planned the subject of study in cooperation with the Belgian Consumers' Association. The data applied only to the Flemish region of the country. Flemish families were used as the base of measurement. 39.1% of all families had used one or more methods of AHC. This would make up a total of approximately 607,420 families. Further analysis of this basic data gives a picture of the individual frequency on an annual basis[11]. Thus, homoeopathy would be used by 8.2% of the adult Flemish population. Acupuncture comes second place (4.3%), followed by manipulative treatments (3.6%), natural remedies (2.8%) and paranormal remedies (2.6%). All other methods scored less than 1% on an annual basis. The data available did not permit patients using more than one form of alternative treatment to be split up. Given a number of hypotheses it is possible to conclude, albeit hesitantly, that the individual extent of consumption of AHC in Flanders would probably lie between 15% and 20%. In 1986, the extent of use of AHC was measured for the first time at a national level and by means of a representative poll[12]. This consisted of an investigation carried out by the Belgian Consumers' Association. The study showed that 31% of the Belgian population aged 15 or older used one or more AHC treatments annually. Homoeopathy was used by 17.5% of the population (11.2% through a practitioner, 6.3% by self-medication). Natural remedies were second with 6.8% (2.4% through a practitioner, 4.4% by self-medication) followed by manipulative treatments with 6.1%, acupuncture with 5.8%, chiropractic with 3.4%, osteopathy with 2.7% and phytotherapy with 2.7%. All other forms took up approximately 1% or less.

With regard to the main areas of symptoms, J Van Hecke noted that many patients made use of alternative treatments for problems with the limbs, muscles and joints[8]. This is especially so in the case of patients of chiropractors. Problems with the stomach, abdomen and digestive system predominated within paranormal therapies. The author points out the marked absence of acute symptoms, infectious diseases, malignant tumours and confinements among the patients of alternative therapists. Approximately 72% of the patients had been suffering for more than one year from their complaints before consulting an alternative practitioner. 85% of those polled had first consulted a general practitioner (where they received treatment by allopathic methods), 56% had first consulted a specialist doctor. According to the patients' own subjective experiences the general practitioners had the lowest success rate. Specialist doctors scored slightly higher and the alternative therapies came out on top. According to the author, most patients visited an alternative practitioner on the advice of friends and acquaintances (lay-referral system) and can be divided into two main categories as follows: the pragmatic who opt for AHC as a last resort and the idealists who reject allopathic medicine as an "incorrect doctrine".

The survey by the Belgian Consumers' Association showed that patients of alternative practitioners have more complaints on average than patients of specialist doctors[13,14]. At the same time patients of AHC have a more negative image of their own state of general health at the moment of starting their own treatment. 44% of the patients of specialist doctors (allopathic) have been suffering from their symptoms for over one year. In patient groups of AHC this figure rises to 68%. Patients of alternative medicine have a longer history of treatment than patients of specialist doctors. They have generally more often been treated by other practitioners previously.

Regarding subjective satisfaction, general practitioners (allopathic) score highest on the extreme positive scores for complaints which can be treated in a single consultation. For symptoms requiring more than one session of treatment specialists score the highest. In both cases it is the case that treatment by alternative therapists is seen to be the best if at the same time less extreme positive judgements are included. Dissatisfaction with the results of treatment within allopathic medicine was the crucial factor which drove patients to try AHC[15]. This factor is seen in conjunction with a certain unease with regard to an over-narrow treatment of complaints (an over-symptomatic approach).

Another element involved is connected with the fact that people are confronted both consciously and unconsciously with the existence of AHC in the world around them. Once the patient has crossed the threshold of AHC, he is more and more attracted and convinced by the absence of iatrogenic effects. In addition the patient is drawn very strongly by the open and comforting relationship with the practitioner and by the fact that the practitioner takes the time to tell the patient about is condition and the proposed treatment.

The availability

Specific research regarding practitioners of AHC in Belgium has been very scarce up to now. This does not mean that there are no facts at all on the availability, even though the data is mainly limited to lists regarding the mainstream educational level of the practitioners.

The survey carried out in 1983 by the Belgian Consumers' Association showed that in the fields of homoepathy and acupuncture, the major share of treatment – 84% and 74% – is carried out by doctors[13]. For homoeopathy, 72% of all treatments are carried out by general practitioners and 12% by specialist doctors. Within acupuncture the figures are 51% by general practitioners and 23% by specialist doctors. In the area of manipulative therapies these figures fall to 20% approximately equally divided between general practitioners and specialist doctors. What is remarkable is that about 12% of patients claim that they have been treated with paranormal therapies by a doctor. Physiotherapists are most strongly represented in the supply of manipulative treatments (33% of all treatments). As regards acupuncture they are responsible for 8% of all treatments and 3% of all homoeopathic treatments. Non-medically or paramedically qualified personnel who use the authority of a specific non-regular course of training to treat patients are mostly found within paranormal (35% of all treatments) and manipulative disciplines (34% of all treatments). Non-medically or paramedically qualified personnel who in addition do not rely on any specific training account for about 52% within the sector of paranormal therapies.

The financial position of alternative medicine in Belgium

AHC is not reimbursed by the Social Security System, whether carried out by a doctor or by a non-medically qualified person. The summary of medical treatments provided does not contain any codes which refer to general or specific technical medical treatments within the area of AHC. Practically speaking, it is possible for doctors practising AHC techniques to guarantee to their patients that part of their professional fees will be reimbursed. The portion that is reimbursed is thus dependant on the grade of specialisation of the doctor and the general and specialist allopathic care to which he refers.

There is a dearth of recent studies into fees charged for AHC treatments in addition to studies into the current methods of repayment. Generally it would seem that there has been no serious research interest in the continued evolution in the financial and economic implications connected with the use of AHC. The only time that financial measures surrounding AHC were discussed in an official report was in connection with the activities of the Royal Commission set up by Statutory Instrument in 1975 with a brief "to propose the most effective methods to reorganise health insurance within the framework of health service management as a whole and to improve its working with reference to cost saving"[16].

The final report of the Petit Royal Commission mentioned AHC in two short remarks. The first time it concerned a statement on the reimbursement of the cost of homoeopathic medicinal specialities[17]. It was stated that such remedies could be reimbursed up until 1950 but after receiving advice from the Belgian Royal Colleges of Medicine they have not been eligible for reimbursement since 1 July 1950. The Petit Commission reported that at the beginning of 1975 both Belgian Royal Colleges of Medicine maintained their viewpoint of 28 February 1950.

The second remark concerned a more precise evaluation of what the Commission referred to as 'new methods of medicine'. This expression was used by the author to refer to homoeopathy, anthroposophy, macrobiotics and acupuncture. According to the Petit Commission there was no evidence to suggest that these forms of treatment would be cheaper in price. The opposite is true, Petit avers; these forms are more expensive when a series of treatments is required.

Based on empirical surveys conducted with patients (both consumers and non-consumers of AHC) and with practitioners (users and non-users of AHC) it would seem that, on the contrary, there is an enormous gulf between the society with its express wish for reimbursement of AHC charges and the relevant authorities, whose attitude is summarised in the Petit Report. The survey carried out in 1983 by the Belgian Consumers' Association shows that only a minority of those questioned think that AHC provided by non-doctors should not be reimbursed[18]. This minority was 13% among patients who have already received AHC treatment, and 21.4% among patients who have never been treated by AHC. To put it another way, not only 87% of all patients receiving AHC but also 79% of patients not receiving AHC would like to see reimbursement for this treatment when it is carried out by competent/certified persons. As in such cases we are talking about reimbursement of treatment carried out by non-doctors, it may be assumed that these percentages would be at least as high for AHC treatment carried out by doctors. In addition it is remarkable to note that 59% of users and 36% of non-users expressed themselves willing to pay higher premiums to cover such reimbursements. Similar results were found in the IIVO survey of 1984[10]. Only 11% of those questioned thought that AHC should not be reimbursed. 28% thought that the treatment was carried out by a doctor. 24% thought that paramedical care using AHC should also be included, whereas 21% laid down as the sole condition for reimbursement that AHC should be reimbursed if carried out by personnel of guaranteed training and experience who are subject to the control of a professional body. 15% of respondents listed no conditions at all. These figures mean that 89% of the population of Flanders is in favour of AHC being included within the Social Fund System. Indeed, 61% want AHC carried out by non-doctors to be reimbursed. The IIVO survey also found that 39% of those in favour of reimbursement were prepared to pay higher contributions for this. A remarkable finding is the fact that three out of four doctors want reimbursement of AHC treatment[19]. Forty-four per cent of doctors can justify such reimbursement only if the treatment is carried out by a qualified 'doctor of medicine, surgery and obstetrics'. On the other hand, 30% would also approve such reimbursements with reference to non-doctors. This last point would apply only to practitioners with a qualification as dentist, pharmacist or paramedic and/or practitioners with guarantees as to their training, experience and membership of a professional body.

Current research on alternative medicine in Belgium
The preceding evidence shows that with a little detective work it is possible to produce a reasonably accurate picture of the social significance of AHC in Belgium. However this picture is in no way complete. It lacks a solid scientific base in many areas. Thus there are more complex and detailed explanations which often have to be based on incomplete or unrepresentative surveys or which must be concluded from approximations based on research, which was not carried out with the intention of permitting specific measurement and analysis based on such measurement. On the other hand there are a number of representative surveys which are, however, too limited in their intentions

and thus provide insufficient opportunities for analysis and interpretation. Also, the representative nature is frequently limited to small non-national areas which does not permit any national conclusions to be drawn. With the exception of these technical and methodological limitations, it is a fact that there is hardly any data regarding practitioners of AHC and their organisations.

These elements. together with the fact that the extent of use of AHC in Belgium must be seen as the highest in Europe[20], are a probable explanation of why the national authorities are showing an interest in setting up a new research project – perhaps also because they are under some social pressure to do so. This will be an extensive research project which will be both a challenge and a promise, as they will link together in a systematic way all the weak or non-existent links which have hampered all previous research regarding AHC in Belgium. The research was set up at the end of 1987 under the sponsorship of the Secretary of State for Public Health and the Disabled. The then Secretary of State, Mrs Wivina Demeester-De Meyer requested that a project be set up to clarify the various social aspects of AHC, taking into account the state of relevant scientific investigation and the research information specific to Belgium. This research project has been awarded to the Faculty of Medicine of the University of Antwerp and will be carried out under the direction of Professor A Herman. This research project will comprise three main areas. The first will consist of a compendium of existing organisations and associations concerned with AHC in Belgium. Emphasis will be laid on their objectives and procedures, in addition to the typology of such organisations as well as to the number of members and the wider social role with reference to AHC, as far as can be ascertained from such bodies. At the same time the organisation will be used to create an input base to quantify the availability of organised alternative practitioners and to show their geographical distribution. A second area is concerned with the alternative practitioners themselves, with the intention of further exploring the characteristics of their personalities and methods of practice and also their treatment and practical matters, which are relevant to their particular profession based on a large number of factors. In the third part the patient takes centre stage. In addition to the compilation a detailed quantitative profile based on consumption of type and scope of AHC, an in depth analysis is envisaged of the motivation and decision-making process which leads to conversion to AHC. A certain amount of time will be devoted to the range of symptoms which lead a patient to request alternative medicine, to his own subjective view of the treatment process in the broadest sense of the term, to the patient-practitioner relationship, and to the personal characteristics of typical users and non-users of AHC. This whole research project intends at last to offer practical relevant findings concerning the parties involved, that is the patients, the alternative practitioners and the policy making area. The report should be completed by Autumn 1990.

References

1. First report of the Central Section of the House of Representatives. In *Pasinomie – Monarchie Constitutionelle* 12 March 1818, pp. 343–346.
2. Huyghe B. Over de Kwaliteitskontrole en de Registratie van Geneesmiddelen in Belgie. Paper presented to the seminar *Therapievrijheid '84*; Antwerp, Rijksuniversitair Centrum, 1984.
3. Sondervorst F A. *Geschiedenis van de Geneeskunde in Belgie.* Woluwe: Elsevier, 1981, pp 161–162.
4. Law of 25 July 1938 tot oprichting van een Orde der Geneesheren. Belgisch Staatsblad, 13 August 1938.

5. Foets M, Nuyens I. *Focus op de Belgische Gezondheidszorg Sociologisch Onderzoeksinstitutuut.* Louven: Katholieke Universiteit, 1980, pp 20–34.

6. *Code van Geneeskundige Plichtenleer.* Opgesteld door de Nationale Raad van de orde van de Geneesheren, Article 34, Brussels, 1975.

7. Van Hecke J. Aard en omvang van niet-officiele geneeskunde in Belgie. *Kultuurleven* 1981; 1: 42.

8. Van Hecke J. De alternatieve genezer. In *Sociologie en Gezondheidszorg: 1,* edited by I Nuyens. Antwerpen-Deventer: VL Slaterus, 1982, p 159.

9. Sermeus G. Alternatieve geneeswijzen: een dubbele dimensie. Paper presented to the seminar *Therapievrijheid '84.* Antwerp: Rijksuniversitair Centrum, 1984.

10. *Het Verbruik van Niet-Officiele Geneeskunde.* Brussels: Interuniversitaire Instituut voor Voorming en Ontwikkeling, 1984, pp 7–9.

11. Sermeus G. *Further Analysis on the Basic Data of the IIVO Study.* Unpublished internal document. Brussels: Belgian Consumers Association, 1985.

12. Sermeus G. *Bekendheid en Gebruik van Alternatieve Geneeswijzen in Belgie Anno 1986. Representatieve Bevraging onder de Belgische Bevolking.* Unpublished internal document (*Test Aankoop*). Brussels: Belgian Consumers Association, 1986.

13. Klassieke geneeskunde en alternatieve geneeswijzen: de ervaring van de patienten. *Test Aankoop* 1983; 245 (Dec): 4–14. (Brussels: Belgian Consumers' Association).

14. Sermeus G. *Rapport Alternatieve Geneeswijzen. Tweede Onderzoeksgedeelte.* Unpublished internal document. (*Test Aankoop*). Brussels: Belgian Consumers Association, 1983, pp 11–20.

15. Sermeus G. *Some Quantitative Considerations on Alternative Health Care in Five European Countries.* An Interim Report Prepared for the World Health Organisation – Regional Office for Europe. Brussels: Belgian Consumers'

Association, 1984, pp 36–39.

16. Royal Decree, 10 March 1975. Belgisch Staatsblad, 13 March 1975. Article 2.

17. Petit J. Verslag over de ziekteverzekering. *Kamer van Volksvertegenwoordigers* 1976; 892 (26 May): 293–416.

18. Sermeus G. Rapport Alternatieve Geneeswijzen. Eerste onderzoeksgedeelte. Unpublished internal document (*Test Aankoop*). Brussels: Belgian Consumers' Association, 1983, p 112–114.

19. Ministerie van de Vlaamse Gemeenschap. Administratie Gezondheidszorg. *Ongepubliceerde Bevraging bij een Representatieve Steekproef van 300 Geneesheren in Vlaanderen.* Brussels, 1986.

20. Sermeus G. *Alternative Medicine in Europe. A Quantitative Comparison of the Use and Knowledge of Alternative Medicine and Patient Profiles in Nine European Countries. Report prepared for the European Commission.* Brussels: Belgian Consumers' Association, 1978, pp 52–58.

CHAPTER 5

Pluralism of medical practice in Germany

David Aldridge

Summary
*A consumer based health service may well be pluralistic;
ie. it will offer modern scientific medicine and complementary medicine. The nature of such complementary
health care provision will vary according to local needs. In
Germany we see health care initiatives which are
dependent upon three factors of availability:*

economic; *according to third party methods of
reimbursement (government or private health insurance),*

cultural; *according to the legal, historical and philosophical traditions of therapeutic freedom ('Therapiefreiheit'), and*

social; *according to community needs.*
*In Germany such a provision is located within a political
context which sponsors initiatives by allocating the
appropriate resources. Consumer based health care is
best delivered in a climate of tolerance and active
collaboration between practitioners, legislators and administrators. Such a climate fosters quality of health care.
(Please note no statistics are available for distribution of
complementary practitioners for Germany. Different disciplines have their own statistics, but there is no forum for
sharing this information.)*

Introduction
There is a tradition of complementary health care in
Germany. Currently, however, consumers are demanding

from their insurance companies recompense for newer forms of health care. This has prompted the insurance companies to demand guidelines from the German government about the recognition of various new practices. In addition, the continuing presence of chronic diseases recalcitrant to modern scientific medical initiatives, particularly cancer, and the claims of some natural medical groups about 'cancer cures', albeit using unvalidated methods, has posed the German government a problem about which therapeutic initiatives to validate. The absence of appropriate methodologies has led to a government sponsored initiative at the University of Witten Herdecke to develop such methodologies, offer guidelines to researchers, and ascertain the extent of non-orthodox cancer treatments. This is, of course, occurring at a time when the EC is implementing legislation for the regulation of complementary medicine, and within Germany itself there is a powerful medical lobby to end the licensing of unconventional practitioners.

Recent discussions about complementary medical practice would suggest that it is incompatible with modern scientific medicine, although some practitioners of family medicine are incorporating alternative medical practices[1,2]. The pragmatics of health care seem to suggest a working compatibility for the delivery of a mixed health care which is missed by theorists.

Throughout Europe there have been varying national initiatives whereby the traditional medicine practices have remained active, albeit informally, and in some cases illegally. Complementary medicine in Europe has grown from the basis of naturopathy, homoeopathy and manipulative techniques. There are also national cultural differences which favour differing approaches. For example, we read that in Finland massage is the most commonly used form of complementary practice and harks back to its roots in traditional medicine[3].

For complementary medicine to flourish there has to be a climate of tolerance and active collaboration rather than restrictive licensing practices. This permissive climate leads to enhanced health care delivery. Such tolerance has been a feature of health care as delivered in Germany[4].

The *Kur*

The *Kur* in Germany exemplifies characteristics of both orthodox and non-orthodox medicine (*unconventionelle Medizin*). Such health care practice is not solely explained by biomedical criteria and is best understood as a social, historical and cultural phenomenon[5,6].

The *Kur* is an institutionalised bathing activity which is also used for health promotion. Naturopathic treatments are used alongside modern bio-medical technology. *Kur* clinics are supervised by qualified orthodox medical practitioners, but also use licensed naturopathic healers (*Heilpraktiker*). The medical directors of such clinics often include some aspect of their own philosophy for therapy. Treatments may include bathing, massage, exercise and dietary considerations.

This mixed approach does not seem too far a cry from what some family practitioners in England have been advocating as avant garde in 'holistic' medicine.

The legislative framework for practising medical alternatives in Germany is permissive. Patients can choose whom to consult; orthodox practitioners, complementary practitioners or naturopathic healders. This situation has developed, not without controversy and vigorous debate, in a philosophical tradition which has tried to understand the basic human condition in health and illness[7]. German Romantic philosophy in the nineteenth century attempted to criticise a natural science which was seen as fracturing nature. The maintenance of health was seen as springing from a unity of mind and body the harmony of the individual with other human beings and a concern for the natural environment.

Again, this does not seem a far cry from our current concerns with environmental pollution, the ravages of modern living and the debate about holistic medicine.

Naturopathic medicine developed into a system of ideas which attempted to reform the dehumanization and excessive curative interventions of some medical practices. To implement these reforming ideas it was necessary to develop economic strategies for public health finance and insurance schemes. these were developed in parallel with a legislative framework which supervised the practice of naturopathic healing, inspected the premises of such healers and licensed practitioners. To qualify as a *Heilprak-tiker* it is necessary to undergo a three year approved training. For medical doctors who so wish to practice, they too must undergo such a course.

It is also important to emphasise that the *Kur* tradition is a part of the tourist industry. For some of these *Kur* activities are reimbursable, either fully or in part, by the insurance companies. In Germany free time bathing, not necessarily swimming as a sporting activity, and sauna, are leisure activities. Health care activity in this system not only belongs to the medical domain, but also belongs to a whole series of diverse activities including diet and leisure. This answers Zola's[8] concern about the medicalization of health care activities. In a way he falls into his own trap by assuming that medicine can take over health care under-standings. Health care in practice is not seen as a separate activity from leisure and living. Given the opportunity of choice, in a suitable cultural context which includes health education, then health activity is inseparable from daily living.

Patients who attend a *Kur* clinic have often been treated in a hospital first. These patients fall into four main groups; patients who need rehabilitation after an accident, patients with a chronic or a serious disease condition, older patients who want to maintain their health and continue working, and those who need a rest cure after retirement. Health care in this approach is not only about promoting well-being in younger patients, which might be considered a luxury, but also keeping older patients fit enough to stay in the employment market.

German medical care incorporates both modern scientific medicine, and the traditional nature-oriented medicine. The curative role of herbal medicines, mineral waters and natural food diets, and the health promotional activities of fresh air and exercise, have remained part of recognised health care activities within the wider culture of German humanism. Complementary medicine, which includes the 'newer' therapies of yoga and acupuncture, is thus part of a continuing tradition of medical pluralism, not a return to traditional methods.

The former situation of East and West Germany shows how economic and socio-political realities effected health care delivery. Both countries had the same historical heritage of *Therapiefreiheit*; "the freedom of a practitioner or patient on the basis of his world view – which always entails a perspective as to the meaning and causation of illness – to select for preventative or curative purposes a mode of therapy which is in conformity with this world view"[4] (p16). Modern legislation in East Germany to prevent the training of *Heilpraktiker*, an emphasis on bio-medical proof of efficacy for treatments, a centrally planned economy, and limited pharmaceutical industry, has meant a restriction in health care alternatives. In West Germany, a liberal market economy, and an acceptance that there was more than one truth in a person's perception of his or her own health, had led to a pluralist health service which could accommodate developing alternatives. This pluralism and therapeutic freedom must be continually defended. In a market economy where health is a commodity delivered by suppliers chasing scant resources then powerful medical organisations will demand that others are not licensed. It is social policy and political will which maintain diversity and freedom in health care, not the market place.

Conclusion

A consumer-based health service may be pluralistic; ie. it will offer modern scientific medicine and complementary medicine. The nature of such a complementary health care provision will vary according to local needs. Local health care initiatives in Europe depend upon three factors of availability:

economic; according to third party methods of reimbursement (government or private health insurance),

cultural; according to the legal, historical and philosophical traditions, and

social; according to community needs. This provision is located within a political context which sponsors initiatives by allocating the appropriate resources. Consumer-based health care is best delivered in a climate of tolerance and active collaboration between practitioners, legislators and administrators. Such a climate fosters quality of health care.

Health care, like the natural world has an ecology. Short-term changes may bring immediate political benefits but without a concern for long-term changes and an overview of the whole system, then continuing damage to communities may occur. Germany has a tradition of tolerant pluralism, which has to be rigorously defended. The general population are vigorous in their pursuit of health care which includes many aspects of self care. Leisure activities are seen as part of carying for one's own health. While the licensing practice for *Heilpraktiker* may be copied as a model for complementary practitioner legislation throughout Europe, it is the less tangible pre-treatment activities within a broader cultural context which may be of most value.

References

1. Fulder S, Monro R. Complementary medicine in the United Kingdom. *Lancet* 1985; 7 Sept: 542–545.
2. Wharton R, Lewith G. Complementary medicine and the general practitioner. *Br Med J* 1986; 7 June: 1498–1500.
3. Vaskilampi T. Culture and folk medicine. In *Folk Medicine and Health Culture: Role of Folk Medicine in Modern Health Care*, edited by T Vaskilampi and C MacCormack. Kuopio, Finland: University of Kuopio, 1982; p2–15.
4. Unschuld P. The issue of structured co-existence of scientific and alternative medical systems: a comparison of East and West German legislation. *Soc Sci Med* 1980; 14B: 15–24.
5. Maretzki T. The *Kur* in West Germany as an interface between naturopathic and allopathic ideologies. *Soc Sci Med* 1987; 24: 1061–1068.
6. Maretzki T, Seidler E. Bio-medicine and naturopathic healing in West Germany. A historical and ethnomedical view of a stormy relationship. *Culture Med Psych* 1985; 9: 383–422.
7. Risse G. "Philosophical" medicine in nineteenth century Germany: an episode in the relations between philosophy and medicine. *J Med Phil* 1976; 1: 72–92.
8. Zola I. In the name of health and illness: on some sociopolitical consequences of medical influence. *Soc Sci Med* 1975; 9: 83–87.

CHAPTER 6

The use of alternative treatments in the Danish adult population

Niels Kr Rasmussen,
Janine Marie Morgall

Summary

Alternative treatment by alternative health practitioners is legal in Denmark. This practice is regulated by the Medical Act which governs the practice of medicine and the law concerning drugs, including natural remedies. This legal approach is founded on the premise that no one shall be hindered in seeking help where they can find it. Non-Danish citizens must reside in Denmark for ten years before they can practise.

Alternative treatments are used in combination with traditional health services, and not instead of those services, although alternative health care is costly. Rather than choosing an alternative treatment because of dissatisfaction with orthodox medicine, patients choose an alternative treatment for a specific illness.

Alternative health care is seen by the population as a legitimate form of treatment. It is only the established professional groups who perceive 'alternative' care as 'alternative' ie. something with which they must compete.

Introduction

In 1987 the Danish Institute for Clinical Epidemiology (DICE) published the results of the first comprehensive national study on the health and morbidity of the adult Danish population[1]. This was a representative study based on interviews with 4753 persons. An important part of the research was to study various aspects of how the Danish population uses the health care system including the alternative health care system.

This article will present results from this survey pertaining to the use of alternative health care as well as selected results from other Danish studies.

In our study we use the term '*alternative treatment*'. A variety of other terms are being used among professionals and among lay people, which reflects the different attitudes to the phenomenon: 'unauthorised treatment', 'non-medical treatment', 'folk medicine', 'untraditional treatment', 'complementary treatment'. None of these terms adequately covers the many different kinds of treatment offered outside the formal health care system.

Since in Denmark a commonly accepted definition as to what is meant by 'alternative treatment' was lacking, our criterion was whether or not the interviewees had themselves paid for the treatment. This distinction is significant in Denmark where national health care services are totally or at least partially free of charge.

What is the status of alternative treatment in Denmark?

Alternative treatments and alternative health practitioners are legal in Denmark. There are, however, two laws regulating and restricting the practice of alternative treatment.

The first law is the 'lægelov' (The Medical Act: law governing the practice of medicine), where there is a special chapter concerning non-authorised health practitioners[2]. According to this legislation it is not illegal for a person to practise alternative health care: however, there are special regulations which govern these non-authorised health practitioners. This legal approach (ie. not forbidding the practice of alternative treatment but regulating its scope) is based on the premise that no one should be hindered in seeking help where they can find it, while at the same time protecting the health status of the general population. This law contains recommendations for the punishment of non-authorised practitioners whose treatment results in danger or damage to the patient.

The law governing the practice of medicine suggests increasingly severe punishments if the practitioner has had a previous offence. Certain treatments are forbidden without the presence of an authorised health care worker (usually a physician). For example, it is punishable by law to treat certain infectious diseases as well as to perform surgery, or administer anaesthesia. In a High Court decision of 1981, acupuncture (when the insertion of the needle breaks the patient's skin) was declared a surgical operation – regardless of the depth of the needle. It is also against the law to use prescription drugs without a prescription, etc.

This section of the Act forbids non-Danish citizens who have resided in Denmark for a period of less than 10 years to practise alternative medicine. It is also against the law to solicit patients through advertising.

The other law affecting alternative treatment is the 'Lægemiddeloven' (The Medicine Act: law on drugs). This law covers the preparation and sale of so-called 'natural remedies' as well as manufactured drugs. For example, it outlines criteria for packaging, patient information and advertising.

In a Danish study of treatment given by 'healers' both healers and patients of healers were interviewed. The conclusion of this study was that legislation in this field is considered sufficient and does not impose limitations on the work of the healers[3].

Other Danish studies

In general there has been very little research done in Denmark on the use and development of alternative health care. In the late 1970s Launse and Jensen did an analysis of primary health care services and alternative health practitioners in a Danish municipality[4]. Through interviews with alternative practitioners and health care workers, they sought to find the answer to why people seek alternative treatment.

The study reports that the persons who use the alternative methods had lost faith in their physicians' treatment and/or had been given up by the physicians. That these patients turned to alternative treatment does not mean they had lost faith in physician care altogether, but rather they had lost faith within the concrete treatment episode. The study concludes that it is a characteristic of those persons who use alternative treatment that they tend to have an overall understanding of the relationship between their health problems and treatment. They therefore claim that they can better understand the treatment they receive from the alternative practitioner than the treatment they receive from their physician.

In a more recent study[5] which asked patients why they had sought alternative treatment, one reason given was that their physician had 'given up on them'. Other reasons included: side-effects of the prescribed drugs: lack of results from the physician's treatment; differences in opinion between the physician and patient as to the cause of the disease; lack of interest from the physician; and the fear of surgery and pain.

In one study conducted at a general practitioners' surgery, over 300 were interviewed about their use of alternative therapy[3]. They found that 41% had sought alternative therapy, women more frequently than men. There were no significant differences with regard to age, social status or diagnosis. Use of alternative treatment was more frequent among the chronically ill. It was the conclusion of the study that alternative treatment was used *in combination with*, and *not instead of*, traditional health services.

In a more recent Danish study on the use of drugs in daily life[7], a questionnaire was administered to members of patient (user) associations. When asked whether or not they used alternative treatments, one third reported that they combined the use of medicine with other forms of treatment. In this study other forms of treatment included physical exercise, special diets and yoga, as well as those which would be classified as more alternative. Less than one quarter reported that they substituted the medicine prescribed by the physician with some other form of treatment.

Table 1

Use of various alternative treatment methods by the Danish adult population 1987

	During the last year %	Ever %
Reflexology	4.2	9.1
Natural medicine (e.g. homoeopathy)	3.6	6.4
Massage/manipulation	2.3	5.2
Relaxation	1.9	3.4
Acupuncture	1.5	2.8
Instructions (on diet exercise etc.)	1.1	1.8
Use apparatus (incl. magnetic passes radioni etc.)	0.6	1.2
Other	1.9	5.0
Percent with one or more of the above	10.00	23.2
No of respondents	4753	4753

Results of the Danish Institute for Clinical Epidemiology Study

What types of alternative treatment are being used by the population?

In our study we sought to determine what types of alternative treatments were being used. Table 1 (see page 87) presents the most frequently used types of alternative treatment methods. No *one* single treatment has been used by more than 10% of the study population. During the last year 10% used one or more of the various treatments, and almost one quarter have at one time or another used one or more methods of alternative treatments.

Who uses alternative health care?

Figure 1 illustrates that it is more common for women than men to use alternative treatment methods. It is most frequent in age groups 24–44 and 45–66. The figures show that the use of alternative treatment has increased as it is becoming more common among the younger generation. No major social differences could be found between users and non-users. The main difference can be found between occupationally active and occupationally non-active (employed vs unemployed). This indicates that alternative health care is costly compared to public health services.

Illness behaviour

In our study we found that during a two-week period more than two-thirds of the population experienced discomfort due to symptoms related to one or more organ systems. one-third experienced extreme discomfort. However, as can be seen in *Figure 2*, many did not respond to the symptoms (40%) while 15% consulted a physician. A fairly large group took previously prescribed medication or used some kind of treatment previously recommended by a physician. Only 2% consulted a provider of alternative care.

Use of alternative treatment among men and women of different age categories 1987

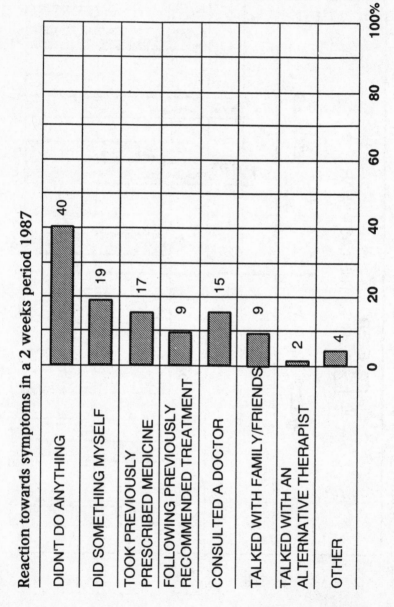

Figure 2.

Reaction towards symptoms in a 2 weeks period 1987

DIDN'T DO ANYTHING	40
DID SOMETHING MYSELF	19
TOOK PREVIOUSLY PRESCRIBED MEDICINE	17
FOLLOWING PREVIOUSLY RECOMMENDED TREATMENT	9
CONSULTED A DOCTOR	15
TALKED WITH FAMILY/FRIENDS	9
TALKED WITH AN ALTERNATIVE THERAPIST	2
OTHER	4

In general, long-term illness appears to be a determining factor with regard to the frequency of physician-contact and use of medicines, whereas it only has a minor (although significant) influence on the extent to which alternative treatment was used (*Figure 3*). Only 13% of those with long-term illness had used alternative treatments during the last year compared to 9% of those without long-term illness.

Table 2 presents the proportion of persons with specific diseases who used alternative care during the last year and compares them with the proportion of those without specific diseases. It can be seen that those having diabetes have used alternative treatment with the same frequency as the population in general, whereas for other diseases the frequency is higher among those with a disease than in the general population. This is the case for men and women having migraine and for men and women with back disorders.

Table 2

Use of alternative treatment among persons with or without selected specific disease.

	Proportion with alternative treatment during the last year	
	Male	Female
Among all	7%	13%
Among those without specific disease	5%	9%
Among those with diabetes	8%	11%
Among those with nervous conditions	7%	20%
Among those with migraine	17%	25%
Among those with back disorder	12%	24%

Figure 3.

Use of family physician, use of medicine and use of alternative treatment in groups with or without long term illness.

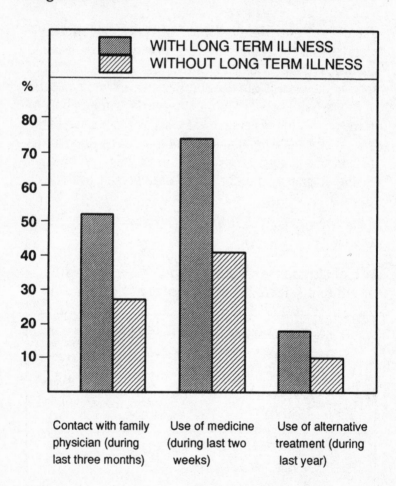

Use of medicines

Figure 4 presents the proportion of men and women who have taken medication during the last 14 days. Large groups have taken analgesics, most frequently women. Only 3% reported have used herbal medicine during the last 14 days.

Figure 4.

Use of various medicines during last 2 weeks 1987

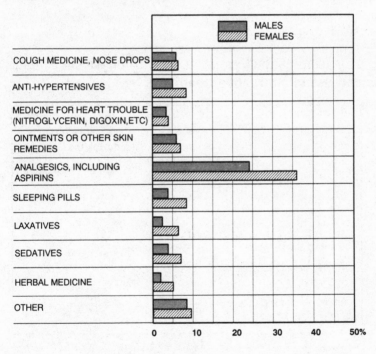

How alternative is the use of alternative treatment?

Table 3 presents the frequency of use of alternative health treatment by men and women who *have not* been in contact with a physician during the last year compared to those who *have* had contact with a physician. In addition, these figures have been compared with the figures for those who are dissatisfied with their physician. The Table displays a very clear tendency: there is a significantly higher proportion of users of alternative treatment among persons who have had contact with a physician. It was especially those women who were dissatisfied with the contact with their physician who used alternative treatment most frequently. This indicates that alternative treatment is not chosen *instead of*, but rather *as a supplement to*, traditional medical treatment.

Table 3

Physician contact, satisfaction with physician contact and use of alternative treatment.

	Proportion with alternative treatment during the last year	
	Male	Female
Among those without physician contact, during the last year	3%	7%
Among those with physician contact, during the last year	8%	14%
Among those dissatisfied with physician contact	12%	29%
Among those satisfied with physician contact	8%	12%

Reasons for choosing alternative treatment
Danish studies report that dissatisfaction with medical treatment, treatment without result, curiosity etc. were decisive factors in the choice of alternative treatment. In our study the respondents were asked (in an open-ended question) what their reasons were for choosing alternative treatment.

Contrary to thse studies our survey found that most frequently the respondents named a specific illness as the reason for seeking alternative treatment. It was seldom reported that an alternative treatment was chosen due to dissatisfaction with or criticism towards traditional medical treatment (*Tables 4–5*).

It has been suggested that the difference between the results in various studies which looked at reasons for choosing alternative treatment can be explained by the very different research settings in which the studies have been performed. it is hypothesised that when a member of the traditional medical system conducts the interviews in a setting in which the respondent is a patient, it might elicit defence mechanisms. The questioning might be perceived as a criticism of the choice of alternative treatment, in which case a natural defence might be to counter the attack by criticising the established system.

Supply and economic implications

A national voluntary organisation which supports alternative treatment methods has compiled a register of therapists: up to now 2500 have registered. In 1978 a local community study found the ratio of alternative therapists to family physicians to be 1:6. For Denmark as a whole this means 2000 alternative therapists. More recent literature reports that, in a Danish municipality with a population of approximately 7000 persons, there were (in 1989) 12 alternative therapists and only seven general practitioners[8].

The amount of money spent on alternative health care varies according to age, sex and socio-economic status, being highest among the elderly, women, and lower-income groups. On average 1300 DKr was spent a year by users of alternative therapists. 320 DKr was spent by users of herbal medicine. In the general population the average

Table 4. **Disease-related reasons for seeking alternative treatment**

	Male					Female					Total
	16–24	25–44	45–66	67+	all	16–24	25–44	45–66	67+	all	
with alternative treatment	14%	18%	20%	19%	18%	19%	31%	32%	21%	27%	22.8%
N	571	1268	964	465	3268	59	1313	978	548	3429	6697
with disease/illness-related reason, hereof diseases of	% 76	% 81	% 84	% 89	% 83	% 78	% 76	% 77	% 83	% 78	% 79.5
– muscular-skeletal system	39	48	51	54	49	32	30	42	47	36	41
– skin	6	6	5	7	6	5	8	4	2	5	5
– nervous system	5	4	4	6	4	7	9	12	5	9	7
– digestive system	1	3	6	6	4	4	4	3	5	4	4
– respiratory system	3	3	3	3	3	7	5	2	4	4	4
– injuries	8	5	4	1	5	2	2	–	3	1	2
– nervous conditions (mental problem)	5	6	4	2	4	3	4	2	2	3	3
N	80	230	192	87	589	110	400	310	116	936	1525

	Male					Female					Total
	16–24	25–44	45–66	67+	all	16–24	25–44	45–66	67+	all	
with alternative treatment	14%	18%	20%	19%	18%	19%	31%	32%	21%	27%	22.8%
N	571	1268	964	465	3268	59	1313	978	548	3429	6697
with non-disease-related reason,	% 31	% 30	% 27	% 25	% 29	% 29	% 35	% 35	% 27	% 33	% 31.3
– dissatisfaction neg. experiences (traditional treatment)	5	10	11	13	10	5	11	9	6	9	9.4
– curiosity	8	6	4	3	5	5	7	6	7	7	6.0
– wellbeing, health promotion	13	10	7	5	9	7	10	11	7	10	9.3
– recommended	4	4	5	5	7	9	5	7	7	6	5.6
N	80	230	192	87	589	10	400	310	116	936	1525

yearly expenditure for authorised medicine was 200–300 Dkr. For the sake of comparison: the average hourly wage for male workers in the Copenhagen area is 120 DKr before tax[10].

Conclusion

Our study supports other findings which show that alternative treatment in Denmark is sought as a supplement to, and not a substitute for, traditional health care. Based on results from our study it might be concluded that alternative health care is perceived by the general population as a natural and legitimate treatment method. It is mainly the various established professional groups, primarily the physicians, who perceive alternative health care as a real alternative, ie. something with which they are forced to compete.

Any health care system which develops and institutionalises treatment methods as established and closed systems (whether presently perceived as alternative or not) will force alternative treatment or innovations to develop outside the system.

From a sociological perspective, 'alternative' treatment could be defined as *non-institutionalised* treatment. In other words, any form of treatment occurring outside of society's major institutions.

References

1. Rasmussen NK, Groth MV, Bredkjaer SR, Madsen M, Kamper-Jmrgensen F. *Sundhed & Syugelighed i Danmark 1987 -en Rapport Fra DIKES Undersmgelse (Health and morbidity in Denmark 1987)*. Copenhagen: Danish Institute for Clinical Epidemiology, 1988.
2. *Betaenkning nr 990 vedr. Naturpraeparater og Ikke-autoiserede Helbredelsemetoder* (Law on natural products

and non-authorized health methods). Copenhagen: Indenrigsministeriet, 1983.

3. Nielsen JN. *Naturlaeger mellem Shamanisme og Videnskab* (Healers – between Shamanism and science). Copenhagen: Munkssgaard, 1988.

4. Launsø L, Jensen HM. *Sundhedsarbedje paa Tvaers* (Health work across the lines). Copenhagen: FADL, 1980.

5. Nielsen JN. Why do patients consult natural healers? *Ugeskr Laeger* 1986; 148: 1780–1782.

6. Dirach J, Kringelbach M, Hansen M, Lund P. Homeopathic medicine, is this an alternative or a supplement to the health services? *Ugeskr Laeger* 1987; 149: 2232–2234.

7. Hansen H, Launsø L, Morgall J. *Samarbejde mellem Brugerorganisationer & Apoteksfarmaceuter om Laegemiddelanvendelse* (Co-operation between patient organizations and pharmacists with regard to the use of drugs). Copenhagen: Institut før Samfundsfarmaci, 1989.

8. Launsø L. Integrated medicine: a challenge to the health care system. *Acta Sociologia* 1989; 32(3).

9. Mikkelsen P, Steenstrup JE. *Brugerbetaling, Prioritering, Styring, Fordeling* (Payment by the user: priorities, control, distribution). Copenhagen: Amternes og Kommunernes Forskningsinstitutet, 1988.

10. Hansen H. *ed. Levevilkar i Danmark – Statistisk Oversight* 1988 (living conditions in Denmark). Copenhagen: Danmarks Statistik og Socialforskningsinstuttet, 1988.

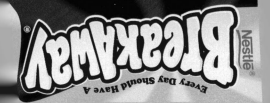

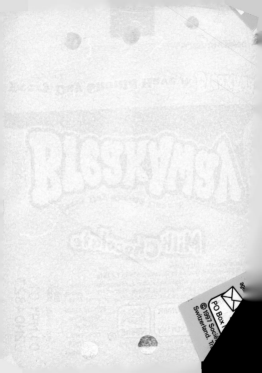

CHAPTER 7

The role of alternative medicine: the Finnish experience

Tuula Vaskilampi

Summary

Finnish law does not recognise alternative medicines. Only medically qualified doctors are allowed to practice medicine, which is interpreted as the right to diagnose and take fees. Acupuncture, however, is accepted as part of orthodox medical practice and is included in the medical curriculum. The field of alternative medicine is heterogenous; there are ancient systems of traditional folk medicine as well as popular alternative medicine ie. manipulative therapies, natural remedies and spiritual healing. Traditional medicines are used by the older, less well-educated rural population. Newer forms of alternative health care are used by a younger urban population. There are no payments from private or public funds for alternative medicine.

Introduction

For alternative medicine to exist as a system it requires a unified official system as a counterpart. From this perspective alternative medicine in Finland, as in other countries, is young. Its origin is related to the emergence of professionalised and legalised scientific medicine which has formed a mandate with the State[1]. The Welfare State has created a public system carrying responsibilities for organising and running health services thereby becoming an agent of social control.

The gap between official and unofficial systems has

grown wider. The union of science and the bureaucratic model of welfare organisation has grown firmer[2]. What has been left outside of this official system has become unofficial and therefore 'alternative'. Alternative medicine as a form of health care is a product of the modern industrial state[3].

It is interesting to note that the practice of acupuncture in Finland is considered as an official form of orthodox health care when practised by qualified medical doctors. Like Canada, Finland was one of the first Western countries to adopt acupuncture into official medicine and acupuncture has been part of the medical school curriculum since the 1970s.

If we consider the Welfare Triangle (see *Figure 1*) we can see the position of different medicines in the relation to

Figure 1.

Different health care systems in the Welfare Triangle

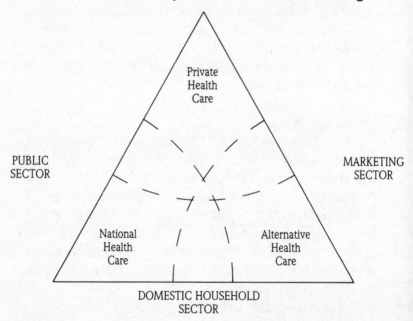

the three main areas of Welfare Society. The supply of official national and private medicine is determined by legal control and financial compensation in the public sector, particularly in the National Health Care system. Private medicine, while controlled by public sector requirements, is influenced by marketing factors. Marketing factors too influence decision making in alternative medicine. This decision making is also influenced by the domestic economy of households.

In Finland National Health Insurance covers both the public and private sectors. Alternative medicine stands outside this system of compensation and also has no legal status.

Finnish legislation regulates and gives the right to practice medicine to medically qualified doctors. The status and role of other health care personnel, and those involved in pharmacy, are regulated by legal norms based on a professional concept of healing practice. Alternative medicine stands outside this legal status although the National Board of Health and Ministry of Health and Social Affairs have expressed an interest in alternative medicine. However, while alternative medicine does not enjoy the support of public policy, it is also free from public restraint.

Folk medicine and popular alternative medicine
The field of alternative medicine is large and heterogenous. It is dynamic and constantly changing. Any definition is temporary. Within the field there are ancient systems of traditional folk medicine as well as modern imports from foreign cultures[3,4,5] (see *Figure 2*). However, with such rapid change, in a context of modernity, some common shared symbolic meanings are being lost.

Finnish alternative medicine can be classified into two main categories:
a) Finnish folk medicine and
b) popular alternative medicine.

Figure 2.

The Roots of Alternative Medicine

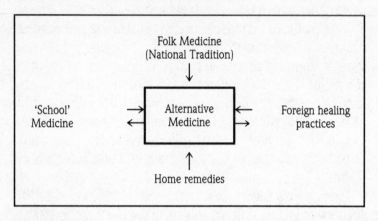

It is important to remember that the boundaries between these categories may be blurred, and that classification systems for alternative medicine are varied[6,7,8]. Within these two broad categories there are sub-categories related to practice.

Finnish folk medicine
1. Manipulative methods: Massage, bone-setting, cupping.
2. Medicines: herbs, alcohol.
3. Naturopathy: sauna, various methods of water treatment.
4. Spiritual and psychosocial approaches: bloodstopping, charlatans, shamanistic healing.
5. Life style advice.

Popular alternative medicine
1. Manipulative methods: chiropractic, osteopathy, naprapathy, zone therapy, lymphatherapy, and assorted therapies.

2. Medicines: natural remedies, homoeopathy, phytotherapy, and natural products.
3. Naturopathy: different forms including 'spas' and 'health farms'.
4. Spiritual healing: different oriental cults, spiritual healers. New 'shamanism', scientism, and various parapsychological schools.
5. Philosophical and doctrinal approaches: oriental philosophies, anthroposophical medicine, theosophical medicine, Ayurvedic medicine and Unani medicine.
6. Psychological and psychosocial methods: psychotherapies, music therapy, dance therapy, art therapy, relaxation therapies (including Yoga and biofeedback).
7. Life style: dietary methods.

These two main forms of alternative medicine differ according to their types of knowledge (empirical or belief system) and learning processes (folk traditional or 'schooled') (see *Figure 3*).

Empirical folk medicines based on natural experiences like cupping, bone setting and massage have long traditions of practice, are not originally Finnish and have a universal knowledge base. These healers are not 'trained' and have not learnt their skills or knowledge from a literature base.

Folk medicines based on belief systems can be seen as supernatural and outside the range of natural laws, eg. blood stopping and shamanism.

Popular alternative medicines are influenced by traditional practice, but they are also influenced by modern scientific discoveries and commercial products. These alternative practices are growing more and more fragmented as practitioners and therapeutic initiatives develop in their own direction.

The use of the term 'Alternative Medicine' in general use is often questioned in Finland, as it can be used in so many different ways. Each therapeutic approach uses

Figure 3.

Examples of Alternative Medicine according to origin and knowledge

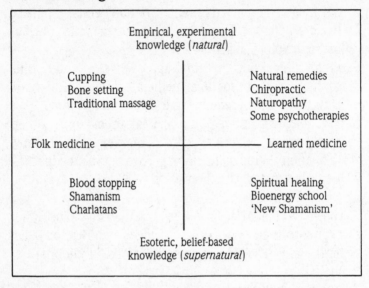

another term according to the concepts underlying that particular practice: holistic medicine, unofficial medicine, natural medicine, organic medicine, folk (traditional) medicine, fringe medicine, physiological medicine. This unstable and rich vocabulary represents a wide variety of dynamic ideas; yet also symbolises different interests and an underlying power struggle.

The doctrines of alternative medicine operate within a different discourse to that of natural science. These discourses are rich and varied in their logic and rationality of disease causation, disease classification, treatment and the assessment of efficacy and therapeutic outcome. Where these views do unite is at the symbolic level outside their concrete manifestations in everyday life[5]. The ideas of alternative medicine have become symbols. The organic is opposed to the mechanical, and consideration of the whole person is opposed to any biomedical reductionism. There is also a stress on vitalism, bioenergy and the self-healing powers of each individual combined with environmental and universal themes.

Research in alternative medicine
There is a long tradition of folk medicine research in Finnish ethnology based on the vast archives of folk lore. This mainly descriptive and historical research has had little influence outside its own field.

In 1978 the Medical Research Council of the Academy of Finland appointed a working group to plan the development of research on physiological treatment methods. On the basis of a report from this group a new group was appointed in 1979 to continue the planning work. Three urgent problems were identified:

1. Research was needed to clarify to what extent physiological treatment methods were used, the reasons for their use and the consequences of their use.
2. Research on the treatment of high/low blood pressure by means of physiological treatments.
3. Research on the treatment of complaints of the neck and back by means of physiological therapeutic methods. Both the working groups used the term physiological treatment, but the underlying concept was that of 'alternative medicine'.

In 1982 a collaborative working group was set up by the Research Council of the Social Sciences of the Academy of Finland to promote research and act as a network of researchers from the different disciplines interested in alternative medicine. The main issues in this work have been the identification of methodological problems, the understanding of different doctrinal positions and the ethical issues involved. There are about 70 people in this collaborative group, and the largest represented disciplines are social science and medicine.

The medical interest has been mainly concerned with the use rates and variability of alternative methods, including what healers exist, their methods and their patients[9]; the motivations of users; the effectiveness of cupping; the use of alternative medicine among cancer patients[10]; and the social structure and effects of vegetarianism.

There is, however, an overall lack of studies on the supply of alternative medicine in the whole country, the economic issues involved and the structure of production. There are very few multi-disciplinary studies and very few experimental studies of the effects of alternative medicine. The University of Kuopio has been active in research, as has the Centre of Folk Medicine in Kaustinen. Kaustinen is based on the idea of combining folk medicine with school medicine where both medically qualified doctors and folk healers (bone setting, cupping and spiritual healing) work in collaboration.

The supply of alternative medicine

There is no general register of practitioners in Finland. There are some organisers and supporters of Alternative Medicine (Association of Organic Medicine, Association of Holistic Medicine, Association of Naturopathy and Natural medicine, and the Association of Health Care Consumers). In 1988 at the Centre of Alternative Medicine in Tampere a ceiling organisation was founded with the aim of co-ordinating the different groups. There are some therapists who remain outside such organisational structures.

There are about 10 chiropractors in Finland and they have been trained in the USA and England. Some therapists train in the School of Alternative Medicine in Sweden but it is impossible to estimate the number. There may be as many as 20 medical doctors practising alternative medicine.

In 1985 a book was published for public use which gave the names and addresses of therapists practising alternative medicine[11]. According to this book there were 659 therapists/healers. The biggest therapist group was zone therapy (30%), followed by bone setters (10%) and spiritual healers (6%). In contrast there are 956 general medical practitioners and 5160 medical specialists in Finland.

The use of alternative medicine

Surveys of the use of alternative medicine date back to the 1970s. Some of these are based on specific demographic groups or disease[10.12], others are based on specific geographical areas[3,5].

The latest survey of yearly usage of health care based on age groups within the population showed that of those using health care 60% had used orthodox medicine only; 32% had used a mixed approach, of which 22% used modern scientific medicine and popular alternative medicine and 10% were heavy' consumers, using all the different forms of available medicine, ie. scientific medicine, doctors' visits, modern drugs, folk medicines and popular alternative medicines[13]. One per cent only were 'pure' alternative medicine users.

Massage is the most used traditional medicine. Natural remedies are the most used popular alternative medicine.

Surveys of alternative medicine users show that between 60% and 80% of those users express their satisfaction. However, most of these expressed satisfaction towards official medicine too. The methods of data collection may influence the results of such studies.

The general trend is that women use alternative medicine more than men. Folk medicine is used by those dwelling in rural areas, low educational level with a low income who are middle aged or elderly. Popular alternative medicine is used by the young and middle aged urban populations. Natural remedies are likely to be used nowadays by those with low levels of education.

However, it is important to point out that there are several subcultures of users, although there are no definite characteristics from the population data.

First there are the health-conscious middle-class middle-aged women who are well educated and innovators of social trends looking for new methods and new life styles. These innovative trends are then transmitted into a broad social pattern of usage.

Second, there are the users of homoeopathic, anthroposophical and some oriental medicines most common among high social class groups.

Third, there are the elderly rural dwellers who use folk medicine. For them medicine is part of their local culture combining shared symbols and belief systems.

Fourth, there are the various new age movements and philosophical approaches. Within this group the belief system associated with health offers a concrete tool for comprehending the world and being active in it in a new way. These descriptions of course are only propositional and not exhaustive.

Conclusion

Alternative medicine is a part of the health care system in Finland. It is at the crossroads of the old and the new, operating in the private territory outside the Welfare State. Alternative medicine offers an alternative health care strategy. Its emergence and consequent publicity have occurred at a time when the Welfare State delivery of health care faces crises of efficiency, legitimacy and cost. When Western industrialised countries move towards the post industrial era their cultures and social structures change, new challenges emerge and new solutions must be sought. Only recently has alternative medicine been recognised by the official system and within the academic field as a factor in this changing field of health care delivery. Despite this recognition, it is still outside the legal system, outside of the system of professionalised training and outside any official organisational structure.

References

1. Freidson E. *Profession of Medicine.* New York: Dodd Mead, 1970.
2. Illich I. *Medical Nemesis.* London: Calder and Boyars, 1975.
3. Vaskilampi T, Merilainen P, Sinkkonen S. Social and individual determinants of the use of alternative medicine in a Finnish population during1982. Unpublished manuscript, 1988.
4. Vaskilampi T. *Strategies of Alternative Medicine in the Finnish Experience. Collected Papers of the Jyväskylä Social Policy seminars.* Jyväskylä; University of Jyväskylä, Dept Social Policy, 1988 (Working paper no. 52).
5. Vaskilampi T. Culture and folk medicine. In *Folk Medicine and Health Culture: Role of Folk Medicine in Modern Health Care. Proceedings of the Nordic Research Symposium,* edited by T Vaskilampi, C McCormack. Kuopio: University of Kuopio, 1982.
6. Fulder S, Monro R. *The Status of Complementary Medicine in the UK.* London: Threshold Foundation, 1981.
7. Inglis B, West R. *The Alternative Health Guide.* London: Dorling Kindersley, 1983.
8. Landy D. *Culture, Disease and Healing: Studies in Medical Anthropology.* New York: Macmillan, 1977.
9. Räsänen O. Hanna the healer. A case study of a Finnish spiritual healer. *Etnologica Scandinavica* 1983; 5: 65–78.
10. Arkko PJ, Arkko BL, Kari-Koskinen O, Taskinen PJ. A survey of unproven cancer remedies and their users in an

out-patient clinic for cancer. *Soc Sci Med* 1980; 14: 511–514.

11. Reponen A, Reponen P. *Parantaja-luettelo.* Helsinki: Tammi, 1985.

12. Vaskilampi T, Hänninen O. Cupping as an indigenous treatment of pain syndromes in the Finnish cultural and social context. *Soc Sci Med* 1982; 16: 1893–1901.

13. Vaskilampi T. Alternative medicine in Finland. Background paper to the European workshop. *The Impact of Non-Orthodox Medicine on Health Care Expenditure.* Utrecht, The Netherlands, 5–7th June, 1989.

CHAPTER 8

Alternative medicine in the Netherlands

Joost Visser

Summary

Orthodox and complementary medicine are integrated in the Netherlands, and this has been actively encouraged by the Government. Clinical and sociological research has been commissioned to provide a basis for policy decisions. Complementary medicines are flourishing in response to public demand, with acupuncture, anthroposophical medicine, homoeopathy, manipulation, naturopathy and paranormal healing the most popular. As in most other European countries, practice is currently restricted to medical doctors with a university training. More women than men visit complementary practitioners, it is generally poorer members of the population who use paranormal healing. The cost of complementary treatments is reimbursed by private and public health insurance when prescribed by a general practitioner. This includes homoeopathic and anthroposophic medicines.

Introduction

As in other European countries, alternative medicine flourishes in the Netherlands. Firstly, its popularity among patients, as measured in the number of visits paid to alternative practitioners, is still increasing. Secondly, although discussion about the theoretical concepts and possible effects continues to exercise many minds, a certain benevolence towards alternative medicine seems to prevail also among regular professionals. A third indication of the relative strong position of alternative medicine is the interest shown by the Government and other relevant institutions. Fourthly, as compared to other countries, research into the field is quite well developed.

The facts and figures to be presented in this paper are mostly based on the results of these research efforts. Together they give an impression of both the importance of alternative medicine in the Dutch health care system and the research undertaken to measure this importance.

The Dutch health care system consists of four echelons, separated by (low) thresholds: the basic (or public health) echelon; the first (or primary care) echelon (general practitioners, social workers, physical therapists, district murses, home helps); the specialist and hospital echelon; the chronic care echelon[1,2]. In this system the general practitioners play an important part. In general, the specialist or hospital echelon may be consulted only on referral by a general practitioner. The same goes for physical therapists, even for those who work in a primary care setting.

Definitions

Alternative medicine is often defined in terms of what it is *not*; namely, as that part of medicine in which one can not have a training nor acquire a title that is officially recognised by the Government. Alternative practitioners themselves use other definitions. According to Aakster, alternative medicine is directed towards the patient as a whole; is promoting health instead of fighting sickness; uses natural, non-harmful forms of therapy; is directed towards restoring balances and strengthening constructive forces; sees the patient as an active participant in regaining health[3]. Since the publication of the final report of the Commission for Alternative Systems of Medicine[4], six 'mainstream systems' are identified: acupuncture, anthro-posophical medicine, homoeopathy, manipulative medicine, naturopathy, and paranormal healing. According to the *Report*, these six share two characteristics. The first is that they differ in their basic assumptions from regular medicine. The second characteristic is more pragmatic in the sense that these six systems are used by a relatively large number of patients.

Out of the different systems that are grouped together as 'manipulative medicine' only chiropractic and osteopathy are 'alternative' in a strict sense. However, these are only rarely practised in the Netherlands. Manipulative therapy is increasingly recognised by the medical profession. The fact that it is still regarded as an alternative system is evident from the difficulties attached to the reimbursement of the cost of treatment.

Legal framework

At the end of the last century, some types of medical practitioners existed. First, there were medical doctors who were trained at one of the Universities. A second group formed those who were trained at what were called Clinical Schools. However, in country areas especially, most help was given by a third group: those who did not have any medical schooling at all.

In 1865 a bill was passed that put an end to this situation. From that time on, the practice of medicine was restricted to medical doctors with a University background. This monopoly still exists. A modification was made only for the paramedical professions, such as physical therapy. In 1964 these professions were simply defined as being 'non-medical' and were given a legal framework on their own[5].

The monopoly of university-trained and qualified practitioners has been a contentious issue over the years. In the late sixties the Government was advised to provide the option for those without formal qualifications to practice medicine, although they were not to carry out specified medical operations. Furthermore, these healers were responsible for possible damage to their patients' health and were not allowed to call themselves 'doctors'. It is this advice that underlies the bill which is to be introduced in parliament in the near future.

Until then, non-medically qualified practitioners are, therefore, formally still trespassing law. However, criminal prosecution is to be undertaken only when the patient's health has been demonstably damaged and a complaint has been lodged with the health inspector. On the other hand, medical doctors are allowed to apply medical techniques, whether these are considered to be alternative or not. The only restriction is the doctors' own disciplinary law, which should prevent them from behaving in contradiction with the standards of the profession.

Within the group of alternative practitioners a distinction can be made between those who are qualified (by virtue of the legal regulations) and those who are capable (by virtue of their training) to practice alternative medicine. All medical doctors belong to the former category, but only part of them to the latter (eg. only those who had any specific training in this field). It follows, therefore, that none of the non-university trained practitioners is qualified, whereas those who graduated from one of the schools for naturopathy can rightly claim ability to practice.

Frequency of use and patients' characteristics

In the last few years some surveys have been held on the frequency of use of alternative medicine[6,7]. In this overview we restrict ourselves to the data that were most recently collected in the Continuous Health Interview Survey of the Dutch Central Office of Statistics.

In 1987 5.2% of the Dutch population visited an alternative practitioner (not his/her own general practitioner); mostly a homoeopath (1.6%), a paranormal healer (1.4%) or an acupuncturist (0.9%). Together, these patients paid approximately 6.5 million visits to these practitioners. To these should be added 7.3% of the population who paid a visit to his/her general practitioner practising alternative medicine (mostly homoeopathy) (6.1 million contracts). Due to overlap between these figures, the total percentage of patients who visited an alternative practitioner in 1987 (whether or not one's own GP) is 11.8%. Together these 1.7 million patients stand for 12.6 million 'alternative' visits. To compare: the number of contracts with (all) general practitioners, medical specialists and physical therapists was estimated in 1986 at 51.1 million, 23.5 million and 29.2 million, respectively[8].

The number of patients who visit an alternative practitioner is still rising (1985: 9.1%, own GPs included). In particular, the number of people who visit their own 'alternative' GP is rising sharply.

More women than men pay a visit to an alternative practitioner (as is also the case with other medical services). Those aged between 30 and 59 are also a little more inclined to visit those practitioners (after the age of 60 the percentage of visitors suddenly drops), and the same applies to people with a higher education and those who are privately insured. Most important, however, is the health: those who visit alternative practitioners feel themselves less healthy than those who do not, and are ill for a relatively long period of time.[9].

The most common complaints to be presented to alternative practitioners are pain in the muscoskeletal system (eg. back pain, stiff neck) and nervous complaints (such as serious headache).

These characteristics and complaints, however, do not fully explain why people take refuge with alternative medicine. A well-known distinction is between those who are frustrated in the regular care, those who go 'alternative' for pragmatic reasons (because it 'might work') and those who opt for alternative medicine out of conviction[10].

Whenever these concepts are used in empirical research, the latter group turns out to be very small[6,11]. Most people try an alternative treatment because they were told that it might help them (by friends or relatives) or because they read about it in a newspaper or magazine. It follows that most patients do not seek alternative help as a substitute to regular help, but as a supplement to it. While being treated by an alternative practitioner, most of them continue to visit their own GP or medical specialist.

This does not mean that all these patients keep their general practitioner informd about their visits. In a recent survey about half of those who visited an alternative practitioner said that their GP knew about these visits[11]. For those who visit a manipulative practitioner the willingness to inform their GP seems to be greater than those who visit a paranormal healer. It might be inferred that patients are well aware of the GP's preferences. While acupuncture, homoeopathy and especially manipulative medicine are increasingly accepted by general practitioners, only very few of them have a positive attitude towards naturopathy and paranormal treatment.[17]

Supply: the number of therapists

The exact number of alternative practitioners in the Netherlands is not known, due to the fact that many practitioners do not belong to any professional association. A survey in 1985 among the organisations of practitioners showed more than 4000 practising alternative professionals: 735 naturopaths, 300 paranormal healers, 220 homoeopaths, 475 anthroposophical professionals (either medical doctors or other professionals, such as anthroposophical nurses), 945 acupuncturists and 1450 manual therapists[12]. About 60% of these organised professionals had a regular education, either as a medical doctor, a physical therapist or a nurse. To compare: the number of general practitioners in the Netherlands in 1987 was 6200, physiotherapists (in a primary care setting) 9000, medical specialists 11,000[8]. The number of non-organised alternative practitioners is not known.

A recent survey among a representative sample of 360 general practitioners showed that almost half of them applied one or more alternative methods, mostly homoeopathy (40%)[11,17]. Only 9%, 4% and 4% of the respondents applied manipulative medicine, acupuncture and naturopathy, respectively. The 'alternative' practices were not very large: the number of patients treated with homoeopathic medicines varied from only 4 to 2000 in every practice (median: 60). Less than 60% of the GPs concerned had any specific training in alternative medicine.

Medical doctors who wish to train in one of the alternative systems can take a part-time course in anthroposophical medicine, acupuncture, homoeopathy or manipulative therapy, lasting from one to four years[13]. Because the title is not legally protected, anybody can call himself a homoeopath or an acupuncturist without having undertaken this specific training. Like medical doctors, physical therapists can also take a (post-graduate) course; most of them qualify for an acupuncture of manipulative therapy.

Without a medical or paramedical training an alternative practitioner-to-be can matriculate in one of the three Academies for Naturopathy offering 3–4 year full-time courses. As can be inferred from the definition of alternative medicine given before, no official status can be derived from the certificate.

Patient satisfaction
Little data is available yet on patient satisfaction. In a 1981 survey among visitors of alternative medicine, 56% of the respondents said that they improved quite a lot, 22% showed some improvement, 22% did not improve at all[6]. Of course these are subjective opinions, and the patients' expectations before treatment had not been measured. It

is interesting to note, though, that these figures do not differ much from those collected in the same survey among visitors of medical specialists. A survey among alternative practitioners' patients in the city of Nijmegen[14] showed much satisfaction. However, a relatively large number of patients were not satisfied with the costs or the results of the treatment and the information given by the practitioner.

Economic implication: financial aspects and reimbursement

The Dutch sick funds, to which some 60% of the population subscribe, have the legal obligation to reimburse all help given by the patient's general practitioner, including homoeopathy and other alternative treatments. Medicines prescribed by the GPs are also reimbursed, but only those which have been registered. As homoeopathic medicines and anthroposophical medicines are excused from registration, their reimbursement is easy. In the future, household remedies that are freely available at the chemist's will no longer be reimbursed by a GP. However, this will not apply to homoeopathic and anthroposophical medicines.

In addition to the legally defined 'standard package' that is the same for all 45 sick funds in the country, each one of them offers a supplementary package to which its clients can voluntarily subscribe. The substance of this package is to be defined by the sick fund itself. In 1988, 26 of the sick funds reimbursed some forms of alternative treatment (mostly homoeopathy, acupuncture and anthroposophical medicine) in addition to the reimbursement given for the GPs' help.

All larger private insurance companies include at least homoeopathy, acupuncture and manipulative therapy, either in their standard package or in a supplementary package. In many cases reimbursement is given only where the practitioner concerned is a medical doctor or a physical therapist, and is a member of the professional organisation[8]. Recently, a new insurance scheme was developed which pays for a broad range of alternative and additional therapies, including those practised by non-medical professionals.

It is not known how much money is spent on alternative medicine each year. Some years ago this amount was valued at 175 to 200 million guilders[6]. (1 guilder equals approximately ½ US Dollar). For 1987 an amount of 400 to 600 million guilders was mentioned[12]. To compare: the cost of the health care system in 1987 was valued at approximately 33 thousand million (extramural health care: 13 thousand million). To estimate the costs of alternative medicine for the health system, the (unknown) possible effects of substitution should be taken into account.

Conclusion

When characterising the Dutch health system in terms of its approach towards alternative medicine[15], it might be called tolerant; although the right to practice medicine is formally reserved to medical doctors, non-medically trained practitioners have almost nothing to fear. Although scieitific medicine forms the core of the system, alternative methods are certainly not totally excluded, as might be the case in more monopolistic systems. In recent years a trend towards integration and interaction between regular and alternative medicine is apparent in spite of the fact that there is little scientific proof of the effects of alternative methods. As indicated in the introduction to this paper this trend can be seen on the level of Government (that installed a State Commission for Alternative Systems of Medicine in 1977) and financial agencies (such as the sick funds), as well as on the level of both medical doctors and patients. The former incorporate (some) alternative practitioners, the latter often combine alternative and regular treatments, given by different practitioners.

Within research into alternative medicine, much of which is financed by the Ministry of Health, two topics stand out. Research into the efficacy of alternative methods (such as manipulative therapy, homoeopathy) is beyond the scope of this paper and shall not be discussed here. Secondly, some research is either performed or planned within the process of interaction and integration and its possible outcomes in terms of costs. In the near future two experiments will be set up (one in a region, one in a health centre) in which general practitioners will co-operate on the basis of a formal agreement. In the evaluation of these experiments the possible effects of this co-operation will be seen. Furthermore, on the ground of a common advice to the State Secretary of Health given by the National Council of Public Health and the Sickness Fund Council, a research programme will be developed into the possible substitution of regular care by alternative care. This programme will consist of studies on, for instance, the consumption pattern of patients and the production, in terms of referring patients and prescribing medicines, of general practitioners who apply alternative methods, versus those who do not[16].

References

1. Doeleman F. The health care system in the Netherlands. *Comm Med* 1980; 2: 46–56.
2. Tiddens HA, Heesters JP, van der Zande JM. Health services in the Netherlands. In *Comparative Health Systems*, edited by MW Raffel. Philadelphia: Pennsylvania State Univ. Press, 1984.
3. Aakster CW. Concepts in alternative medicine. *Soc Sci Med* 1986; 22(2): 265–273.

4. Alternative medicine in the Netherlands: summary of the report of the Commission for Alternative Systems of Medicine. In *Report of the BMA Board of Science Working Party on Alternative Therapy.* London: British Medical Association, 1986.

5. Kortenhoeven D. *Verboden Toegang voor Onbevoegden.* Utrecht: National Institute of General Practitioners, 1982.

6. Ooinjendijk WTM, Mackenbach JP, Limberger HHB. *Wat Heet Beter?* Leiden: Nederlands Instituut voor Praeventieve Gezondheidszorg/TNO, 1980.

7. van Sonsbeek JLA. Het raadplegen van alternatieve genezers en huisartsen in 1985–1987 (with summary in English). *Maandbericht Gezondheidsstatistiek (CBS)* 1988; 7(8/9): 4–13.

8. Kuindewrsma P, Peters L. Haalbaarheid experimentele samenwerkingsverbanden van huisartsen en alternatieve generzers. Utrecht: NIVEL, 1988.

9. van Sonsbeek JLA. Het raadplegen van alternatieve genezers in 1979 in 1981. *Tijdschrift Sociale Gezondheidszorg* 1983; 61(15): 506–514.

10. Aakster CW. Patiënten-motieven en niet officiële genezers. *Nederlands Tijdschrift Geneeskunde* 1975; (42): 1611–1616.

11. Visser GJ. *Huisartsen en Alternatieve Geneeswijzen; een Onderzoek naar Meningen en Ervaringen van Huisartsen en Patiënten.* Utrecht: NIVEL, 1988.

12. Maasen van den Brink H. *De kwantitatieve Betekenis van de Alternatieve Geneeswijzen in de Jaren Tachtig.* Noetermeer: Nationale Raad voor de Volksgezondheid. 1987.

13. van Es JC. Conventional medicine and complementary therapies in the Netherlands: patterns of collaboration. In *Talking Health,* edited by Sir James Watt. London: Royal Society of Medicine, 1988.

14. Fleuren M, Schouwink I. *Ervaringen van Gebruikers*

van Alternatieve Geneeswijzen. Nijmegen: IBAG, 1988.
15. Jingfeng C. Toward a comprehensive evaluation of alternative medicine. *Soc Sci Med* 1987; 25(6): 659–667.
16. *Advies Mogelijkheden Onderzoek van Substitutieeffecten/Verzekerbaarheid Alternatieve Geneeswijzen.* Zoetermeer: Nationale Raad voor de Volksgezondheid, 1988.
17. Visser GJ, Peters L. Alternative medicine and general practitioners in the Netherlands. *Family practice* 1990; 7(3): 227–232.

CHAPTER 9

Non-orthodox health care in the UK

Kate J Thomas

Summary

Non-orthodox health care (that which does not have official recognition and is practised largely outside the National Health Service) is growing in popularity in the UK. There is no legal prohibition of practice by non-medically qualified practitioners who provide the largest proportion of non-orthodox health care to the public. Compared with orthodox primary care, there are fewer children and elderly patients attending practitioners of the most popular non-orthodox therapies, but a similarly high proportion of women use both types of care. The majority of patients appear to use non-orthodox care as a supplement to, rather than a substitute for, orthodox care.

Definitions, or what's in a name?

In the UK, the use of health care interventions which are not strictly bio-medically based or allopathic in their approach both pre-dates modern medicine, and has continued throughout this century.

The way in which such modes of care are defined and labelled has a history of its own. In post-war Britain it is possible to trace the changing terminology in academic and media output through a number of changes. In the 1960s and early '70s the rather perjorative term 'fringe' was popular as in Brian Inglis' book *Fringe Medicine*[1]. By the late 1970s, the same author was redefining the area as 'natural medicine' and, at the same time, the term 'alternative' medicine became more widely used[2]. Even more recently the terms 'holistic' and 'complementary' have come into common usage.

While each of these terms defies precise definition, such labels are useful as indicators both of the status of this form of health care and of its relationship to orthodox care. 'Natural' and 'holistic' are both terms which attempt to unify disparate therapies and disciplines by an implicit contrast with aspects of orthodox medical practice. 'Natural' conveys a message of procedures of non-invasive therapies in contrast to the chemotherapeutic and surgical procedures of orthodox medicine, while 'holistic' taps the idea of a patient as an integrated psychological and physical entity, located firmly in a social context. This is in direct contrast to the perceived reduction of people to symptoms or diagnoses within orthodox nosologies. These implicit value judgements were challenged in the report on alternative therapies published in 1986 by the British Medical Association[3]. In this report, these implied criticisms of orthodox medicine were represented both as being a cause for concern and, at the same time, falsely based.

The terms 'fringe', 'alternative' and 'complementary' have a different relationship to each other, and to orthodox medicine. Each term may be seen as reflecting a physical relationship to the *practice* rather than the *content* of orthodox medical care. In this typology, 'fringe' medicine is seen as being so far removed from the orthodox, and such a minority pursuit, that it has no effect on mainstream events. Moving along an imaginary continuum, 'alternative' medicine suggests less of a minority activity and somewhat more of a challenge to the majority practice; the latter has become, to some extent, 'optional'. Finally, 'complementary' medicine moves even further along the imaginary continuum of interaction; towards acceptance from one perspective, or incorporation from another. A growth of interest in alternative techniques and philosophies by orthodox medical practitioners has been documented[4,5,6]; this may indicate that the future of non-orthodox care in this country lies more in its incorporation into orthodox practice than in its attainment of independent acceptance and freedom to develop as a parallel practice. As a professional strategy, incorporation has a proven history[7]. In the UK today, the struggle between 'alternative' and 'complementary' has not been resolved at either the ideological or the practical level. In the meantime, whilst no doubt laying myself open to criticism, I will refer to these practices as 'non-orthodox'. The presence or absence of state legitimization is an important distinction, although it must be acknowledged that non-orthodox medicine in the UK has survived, even thrived, with very little official recognition to date.

Legal constraints and freedoms

Alternative health care in the UK today is available from two distinct groups of practitioners: those who have an orthodox medical training and those who do not. Unlike most other European countries, it is not illegal for someone without orthodox medical qualifications or any form of state registration (such as the status of a profession allied to medicine) to offer therapeutic care to members of the public on a professional (fee paying) basis. Some non-orthodox practitioners (osteopaths) are actively seeking State recognition, but the right to practise without formal recognition is established in British Common Law. This protects an individual's freedom to carry out those activities not specifically prescribed by an Act of Parliament. However, within this framework of relative freedom to practice, certain controls are enforced. Proscribed activities include advertising a treatment as a cure for cancer, diabetes, epilepsy and tuberculosis. Non-medically qualified practitioners are also restricted in the titles which they may use, and the commercial use of the term 'health centre' in relation to any premises where doctors and nurses are not employed is prohibited by law. In 1989, the conferment of degree titles and their usage was restricted to recognised institutions which currently include only two of the training centres for alternative practitioners.

These relatively non-restrictive conditions are currently under threat from European Community Law which may result in the situation in Britain becoming more like that in other EC countries, where greater legal controls apply. However, in the past two decades non-orthodox health care appears to have flourished in the UK, to the point where most towns of a reasonable size might now be expected to have some form of alternative health care on offer to the public.

Practitioners

Practitioners of non-orthodox health care in the UK do not form a homogeneous group. The first distinction has already been made between those with orthodox medical qualifications and those without. Estimates made in 1981 suggest that access to non-orthodox care is largely through non-medically qualified practitioners with the latter out-numbering medically qualified practitioners by a ratio of at least 12:1[8]. More recent reseach suggests that there is an increasing interest in the practice of non-orthodox techniques amongst orthodox medical practitioners[4,6]. However, many orthodox medical practitioners with training in a therapy such as homoeopathy will be using the technique in only a minority of their consultations[9].

Precise data on the nature of training in non-orthodox therapies received by orthodox medical practitioners is not available, but many of the courses on offer to such doctors appear to be of a relatively short duration, designed to impart limited skills.

Those practitioners engaged in non-orthodox health care who do not possess an orthodox medical qualification are also a mixed group. Estimates of supply in the UK are notoriously unreliable as there is no registration scheme or centrally held directory of such people.

Practitioners may range from people who have undergone a three year full-time course, who earn a living by practising full-time and charging professional fees, to those who have minimal training or even claim to possess a healing 'gift'. These practitioners may practise part-time, occasionally, or rarely, and some, especially spiritual healers, may not make any charge for their services.

For those disciplines or therapies where full-time or extensive part-time training is available to practitioners, for example acupuncture, chiropractic, homoeopathy, naturopathy, and osteopathy, it is also possible to identify professional associations which serve to guarantee minimum training standards and impose a code of ethics on their members. However, these associations do not act as a formal legal register and it is not always possible for members of the public accurately to identify the status of a practitioner. Ultimately patients must rely on word-of-mouth recommendations as a means of selecting practitioners.

A recently completed national survey suggests that, in 1987, the population of non-medical practitioners who belonged to a professional association and actively practised acupuncture, homoeopathy, medical herbalism, chiropractic, osteopathy or naturopathy in the UK, was in the region of 2,000[10]. This sub-set of non-orthodox practitioners are likely to form the majority of practitioners who would be affected by any proposal to introduce state registration or the protection of titles in the next decade. The same study found wide geographical variations in the supply of these practitioners in Britain. Many practised from more than one location and the majority of these locations (70%) were found in the south or south west of England, more than a quarter were located in the Greater

London area. This distribution mirrors both National Health Service (NHS) provision and private health care facilities in Britain[11]. The majority of practitioners in the study were manipulative therapists. Chiropractic and osteopathy were available at more than half the locations, acupuncture at a quarter. No important regional differences were found in the geographical distribution of therapies available. Large variations were, however, found in the number of consultations per week reported by the practitioners according to the type of therapy they offered, ranging from a mean of 82 consultations per week (SD 40) for the chiropractors to 25 per week (SD 24) for the homoeopaths.

Practitioners' reports of their total weekly workload indicated that an about four million consultations were undertaken in 1987. Regional variations in consultation numbers reflect the distribution of supply. Nationally, four million consultations would represent one consultation for every 55 NHS general practice (GP) consultations, but in Greater London the ratio would be one non-orthodox consultation for approximately 25 NHS GP consultations.

Patients
Studies estimating the level of utilisation via population surveys suggests that anything up to 14% of the population may have used non-orthodox health care at some time[12]. However, these estimates are likely to place non-orthodox health care in the field of self care and include behaviour such as over-the-counter purchasing of herbal remedies in the estimates. People who have purchased vitamin or mineral supplements may be quite different from those who have sought consultations and treatments with non-orthodox practitioners; the relative costs to the patients are also likely to be very different.

There exists comparatively little in the way of representative data on the people who use non-orthodox health care in Britain. The popular stereo-type of these patients is that they are middle class, middle-aged and female. One study of practitioners' impressions of their patients reported that 66% of patients were thought to be female, 30% aged between 41 years and 60 years, and 64% were thought to be from professional or managerial occupations or students[13].

The study by Thomas *et al* which focused on the patients of non-medically qualified acupuncturists, chiropractors, osteopaths, naturopaths and homoeopaths, registered with a professional association, also found evidence to support the popular image of patients; 63% of patients were found to be female, and an estimated 46% were aged between 35 years and 54 years. Three quarters of patients reported non-manual occupations. However, it should be remembered that a similar proportion of NHS GP consultations are with women[14] and, while the elderly are considerably underpresented as compared with patients in NHS general practice, the study estimates that 15% of non-orthodox patients are aged 65 or over[10].

Conclusion

Issues of efficacy continue to be raised regarding non-orthodox medicine in Britain, but relatively little funding is available to pursue such research. In the meantime, members of the public are voting with their feet and using non-orthodox health care at considerable expense to themselves in a country where primary health care is largely free at the point of delivery. The middle-aged, middle-class secton of the population are at the same time more likely to have disposable income to spend on health and less likely to receive free prescribed medication from orthodox practitioners. It could be that they are choosing to spend their money on an alternative form of health care. There is much speculation, but little evidence, on the reasons why people choose non-orthodox health care in Britain today. Recent research[10] suggests that, in Britain in the late 1980s, patients' use of non-orthodox health care should be seen more as a supplement to orthodox care and less as an alternative. patients appear to be selecting what they believe they need from each system independently. The implications of this for effective health care are as yet unclear[15].

References
1. Inglis B. *Fringe Medicine.* London: Collins, 1964
2. Inglis B. *Natural Medicine.* London: Collins, 1979
3. British Medical Association. *Report of the Board of Education and Science: Alternative Therapy.* London: BMA, 1986
4. Wharton R, Lewith G. Complementary medicine and the general practitioner. *Br Med J* 1986: 292: 1498–1500
5. Reilly D T. Young doctors' views on alternative medicine. *Br Med J* 1983; 287: 337–339
6. Anderson E, Anderson P. General practitioners and alternative medicine. *J Roy Coll Gen Pract* 1987; 35: 52–55
7. Johnston T J. *Professions and Power.* London: Macmillan, 1972
8. Fulder S, Monro R. *The Status of Complementary Medicine in the United Kingdom.* London: Threshold Foundation, 1981
9. Swayne J. Survey of the use of homoeopathic medicine in the UK health system. *J Roy Coll Gen Pract* 1989; 35: 503–507.
10. Thomas K J, Carr J, Williams B T. The utilisation of alternative health care systems in relation to orthodox medicine. Unpublished report to Nuffield Provincial Hospitals Trust, 1990
11. Nichol J P, Beeby N R, Williams B T. Role of the private sector in elective surgery in England and Wales,

1986. *Br Med J* 1989; 298: 243–247

12. Consumers Association. Complementary medicine. *Which?* 1986; October: 443–447

13. Fulder S, Monro R. Complementary medicine in the United Kingdom: patients, practitioners and consultations. *Lancet* 1985; 7 Sept: 542–545

14. OPCS. *General Household Survey 1986.* London: HMSO, 1989

15. Murray J, Shepherd S. Alternative or additional medicine? A new dilemma for the doctor. *J Roy Coll Gen Pract* 1988: 38: 511–514

Evolving problems for natural medicines within the European Community – and the biocentric practitioners who use them

Harald Gaier

Summary

European harmonisation efforts lead to 'directives' for general legislative changes, about which confusion often exists. This is partly so because EC member states occasionally obstruct that process of change. Because UK civil servants in Brussels seem to fail to report back to British interest groups and politicians, general ignorance about developments in the European Commission is widespread in the UK. By contrast, some of those who lobby in Brussels and Strasbourg for their special concerns appear to be rewarded for their efforts. The present stage of development, in what is still a very fluid situation, appears to be:

1. The criteria for clinical trials have not been established yet, though it seems that there is to be some flexibility to accommodate the biocentric medical paradigm.
2. There is inconsistency in the draft regulations surrounding injectables.
3. Low potency and unpotentised 'simplexes' for self-medication are now a part of the cultural heritage of Europe and might be proscribed by the bureaucracy at its peril.

4. The future practice of homoeopathy in the classical sense seems to be quite safe and will not be tampered with.

5. Most complex remedies with components of potency levels below 6D seem destined to disappear.

6. Single homoeopathic prescriptions in low potencies will remain available to all practitioners.

7. Oral and external complex remedies with all components above the 6D potency limit will be classified as 'specifics' that have to undergo clinical trials if they are to be sold 'OTC' (over the counter) or on a 'pharmacist's prescription', but would be offered a simplified registration procedure if sales are restricted to 'only on practitioner's prescription'.

8. The UK Government evidently officially recognises the principle of plurality of choice in medicine and in therapeutics, but in other countries this is much more fully developed.

9. Changing all potencies upward beyond the 6D limit in 'complexes' will mean, for the practitioners who use these, getting used to completely changed responses in patients.

10. Registration in two EC countries will probably mean an automatic pan-EC registration for a product.

11. The UK Government will possibly soon want to insist on properly defined professional categories of non-orthodox practitioners with adequate academic grounding, to distinguish them from lay persons, not least because the homoeopathic pharmacists may soon need to have a firm basis for such a distinction.

12. There are several unresolved issues that require attention on an international level without delay.

The backdrop

The familiar 1957 Treaty of Rome and, in the UK, the Single European Act (of December 1985) set the stage for the progressive abolition of trade restraints among the EC member states. This is preparatory to the establishment by 31 December 1992 of a unitary European mega-market, which comprises 335 million inhabitants, many of whom are financially quite well-endowed. Though it has so often been promised by many, it has proved impossible to keep all political aspects segregated from the accompanying intra-European streamlining of economies, finance and trade. It is in the nature of this massive compulsory conversion to near-uniformity, euphemistically termed 'harmonisation', that a large volume of legislation constantly needs to be generated. This, though primarily designed to establish uniform trading rules, inevitably profoundly affects adjacent areas of human interaction. It is sometimes seen to be a pettifogging process of growing together by the 12 participant states into what many hope – some say, naively so – could soon become a United States of Europe.

The evolutionary procedure for this so-called harmonisation is that consultations at various earlier stages can take place between interested parties and the Brussels bureaucratic machinery, before a *Directive* is finally produced by the European Commission in Brussels. Once this gestative process has begun, it becomes an extremely complex, rigidly formalised progression of events, clouded by overwhelming bureaucratic impediments to any normal decision-making processes. In fact, intervention for the purpose of initiating amendments is often said to be arduous to the point of virtual hopelessness. Yet there are, it seems clear, some parties who have more 'equal' access than others to those who ultimately decide. It will surprise no-one that lobbying, or some might say influence-peddling, is political currency in both Brussels and Strasbourg. Hence it appears consistent with the evidence that very powerful special-interest groups, working as inconspicuously as possible, might dispose over a great deal of purchase in areas that could affect the pharmaceutical domain, such as homoeopathy.

It is curiously unconsoling to learn from the legal specialist on the management committee of the All-Party Parliamentary Group for Complementary and Alternative Medicine that "unlike other EC members, the British Government has declined to be involved officially in this process (the negotiations over details of the selection, preparation and formulation of homoeopathic medicines), claiming that to do so is a wasteful "diversion of effort and because of the need for economy"[1]. And it is downright chilling to be confronted by the same man with the allegation that British interests are often simply ignored in Brussels. The reason for this, he maintains, is that whereas the British government has its civil servants in place on many EC bodies at all levels, these – reluctant to admit that their powers are now curtailed – generally fail to consult both their political masters, the ministers, and the relevant interest groups in the UK[2].

A *Directive* that eventually results then requires the national legislatures of the states to pass laws in all their respective countries to implement its injunctions. There are certain safeguards for the purpose of restraining EC states from adopting laws in conflict with existing or prospective *Directives*, but these are periodically flouted.

The dissenters

A case in point is the latest proposed *Directive* relative to the availability of homoeopathic medicines (refer to *SYN 251* dated 28.3.1990), which dovetails with two earlier *Directives (65/65 EC* and *75/319 EC)*, by covering broad areas adjacent to them. The latest one specifically states (in Article 7) that a simplified registration procedure for homoeopathic preparations ought now only to apply to homoeopathic medications for oral or external application provided that [constituents of] such medicines are also chemically more dilute than one part per million. To clarify that, it should be noted that 6D (=6x) of a single medicine, on its own, is the approximate homoeopathic equivalent of 1ppm depending, of course, on the concentration of the pharmaceutical substance in the mother tincture. To complicate matters a little, it must be added that when this medicine is part of a combination, the other constituents act as further diluents themselves. Thus, although a chemical dilution greater than 1ppm is stipulated in the *Directive*, 6D would, in practice, prove to be the acceptable lower limit. That means oral as well as external remedies containing potencies lower than 6D, but all suppositories and injectables or other parenterals would utlimately need to go down the arduous and very costly road of fully establishing safety, quality and efficacy. It is the last of these, the claims to efficacy, that causes most of the difficulties, as will be discussed later.

Moreover, Article 4 of another draft *Directive* (refer to SYN 230 dated 20.1.1990), relating to patient-delivery of non-veterinary medicines, proposes to restrict all parenterals (that includes injectables) as becoming subject henceforth to an orthodox medical practitioner's prescription before becoming available to the patient.

In direct conflict with this, one of Germany's Federated States (North Rhine-Westphalia) passed a statute (on 11 August 1989) *Richtlinien fuer die Ueberpruefung von Heilpraktikeranwaertern*, gazetted 18.9.1989, vol 50, p 1179) which in paragraph 3.1.2 incorporates 'injection techniques' into the prescribed state examination curriculum of naturopaths.

More or less contemporaneously, in another instance, Italy has pre-emptively veered in the opposite direction by passing a law that quite simply outlaws all sarcodes, sarcode-derivatives, isopathics and nosodes, at whatever potency. Additionally, all other homoeopathic medicines, if these are below the 6D potency (for instance, Schlussler's

Tissue Salts are commonly in the 6D range, and sometimes a little below). This is clearly in conflict with much of *Directive SYN 251*, particularly Article 6, as will be explained.

To highlight the divergency in the different official attitudes by the various Governments, it is interesting to note that Denmark, for example, is apparently quite rigidly set against any legislation that would favour homoeopathy, even though all practitioners appear to be as free as they are in Britiain to practice it there. It appears to be contradictory, yet it ceases to be incomprehensible when one hears the rumour that the lobbying by entrenched conservative elements in orthodox medicine, and by some vested-interest groups in pharmaceuticals, has been surprisingly successful in Copenhagen.

Discussion

Some issues that arise out of the said draft *Directives* and out of related matters resulting from the European harmonisation effort are discussed in the next section in a little more detail. The possibly distant prospect must be borne in mind that there may still be significant radical changes to the draft *Directives* which could, perhaps, alter matters dramatically.

Randomised trials not absolutely necessary

The *Directive* of January 1985 (*65/65 EC*) stated that the results of medical and clinical trials are required to establish efficacy and safety. Although the *Directive of May 1975* (*75/319 EC*) defined clinical trials as randomised therapeutic comparisons, it goes on to state expressly that non-randomised medical investigations may likewise be presented. Happily, some of the investigative models proposed from time to time by various authors in the journal *Complementary Medical Research* would, it now seems to the author, be perfectly acceptable in law. Other opinion has it that the criteria for clinical trials in homoeopathy have simply not yet been determined.

The non-sequitur of regulations surrounding injectables
The stipulation that would have all parenteral medication on 'prescription only' by medical practitioners, which would include homoeopathic injections above 6D, does not make much sense. Beyond 8D (this happens to be the standard lithotherapeutic injection potency commonly in use in France, for instance) all injectables are safe in the hands of those properly trained to administer injections. In any chemical sense they are virtually devoid of medicinal substance, ie. they could be viewed as simple physiological saline. Consequently, safety cannot be an issue. If the issue, on reflection, turns out to be the homoeopathic quality of these products, or the standards of sterility and hygiene during their manufacture, then one would have thought control methods to assure adherence to pharmaco-poeial standards and to the rules of contamination-free production methods, by manufacturers rather than con-trols over those who administer the injections, would need to be addressed by the *Directive*. Moreover, many injections are absolutely safe in potencies below the 8D range also.

In its paradoxical restrictions this draft *Directive* would appear to have the effect of furthering the spread of a medical monoculture in Europe. In the UK it means that, although the naturopaths and other practitioners who, with proof of proper training in the technique of adminis-tering injections, are perfectly entitled to do so, the material to be injected (whether nosode, homoeopathic and vitamin injectables) could now be arbitrarily withheld from them. That would represent, to the writer, an unwarranted restriction in the established mode of practice of certain practitioners, while being of questionable value overall.

Another aspect here is the apparent blurring of any distinction between form and essence of a medicine. Surely the process of registering a medicine needs to revolve around the assessment of the particular medicinal substance and its effects on a patient, and not around the presenting form of that medicine. This distinction is in danger of becoming obscured in these draft *Directives.*

Does a grey market in low potencies loom?

Many practitioners in every EC country use anthroposophic, biochemic and homoeopathic medicines somewhere in the range from mother tincture to 6D, as well as higher – occasionally much higher. Additionally, almost all combination remedies have most or all their components in that low potency range, which means most of such remedies could disappear, not because they are not effective, nor because they are unsafe, nor because there is anything amiss with the product's quality, but because the manufacturer simply does not have the astronomical sums of money that would be required to pay for the batteries of controlled clinical trials to prove that these well-established, sometimes centuries-old remedies, are what many already claim them to be, namely neither ineffective nor unsafe. Their commercial success as 'over-the-counter' or 'pharmacist's prescription' medicines can be taken to corroborate that. Is it scurrilous to pose the question whether it is precisely this evident commercial success which has generated the present official inurement that their manufacturers must prove their safety, quality and efficacy by clinical trials?

These medicines are perceived by the peoples of Europe as part of the folk medicine of the last two hundred years and as such they form part of Europe's cultural heritage – particularly in France and Germany, and to a far lesser extent in the UK. If potencies of below 6D were to disappear, as some now fear, it seems a safe bet that a grey market in these remedies, quite beyond the control of any hidebound regimenter, would immediately flourish. After all, every homoeopath since Hahnemann holds fast to the historical right as practitioner to prepare all the necessary remedies for his patients whenever that need arises. On all the past occasions when officialdom was manipulated by the apothecaries to enact similar restrictive legislation against the homoeopaths that is what happened.

With these *Directives* a mildly grotesque situation has developed for the Germans. Their naturopaths (*Heilprak-tiker*) and medical practitioners who practise in the same way have until now worked with an officially sanctioned safety limit much below the 1ppm level, namely at the 3D potency level. If one bears in mind that a homeopathic mother tincture is one tenth of the strength of a phytotherapeutic or allopathic tincture of like name, then a 3D potency represents a chemical deconcentration of the original substance amounting to at least one in 10,000. The potency levels in the combination remedies and of single remedies widely in use in Germany are obviously adapted to this, and practically no investigative work to establish safety at potency levels between 3D and 6D has been undertaken because, in the past, there was no perceived need. Is it that, whatever work in this area was done by all the Germans, which is thought to be considerable, could now all be rendered irrelevant in practical terms by the stroke of a Brussels pen?

What of combination remedies ('homoeopathic complexes')?

A combination remedy, which is acknowledged as being "within the scope and tenets of Homoeopathy" by the *Homoeopathic Pharmacopoeia* of the United States[3] is created whenever at least two distinct substances are mixed together in a set proportion to the whole, after the constituent medicinal components were separately potentised (whenever these are not added as mother tinctures). The homoeopathic medicines are combined in a specific way and normally mass produced in order to target them at specific disease entities. It means at the very least that there is an implicit claim being made for the efficacy of the combination by the manufacturer. Therefore, in that sense it is a pharmaceutical specific. Legislation worldwide is tending toward requiring the producers of all specifics, and of such 'homoeopathic' combinations even if only identified by numbers, to submit them to clinical trials to substantiate their explicit or implicit claims. This process, for which the standards are very exacting, is extremely costly and fraught with numerous difficulties. Hence, it seems possible that many of the combination remedies now freely available over the pharmacy counters in Britain, France, Germany and elsewhere, may disappear in their present form during the last decade of the twentieth century.

The *Homoeopathic Pharmacopeia* of the US notwithstanding, the abiding impression haunting many homoeopaths is that in prescribing a combination remedy (or a so-called 'homoeopathic complex') the prescriber should be betraying his-her fundamental commitment to homoeopathy, because there can never be proper individualisation of a case as homoeopathy requires. Nonetheless, the question remains whether it would not be better for some individual to self-medicate for 'flu-like conditions with an intrinsically harmless 'homoeopathic' combination that made unsubstantiated claims, rather than with, say, phenacetin, paracetamol or aspirin, with the real risk of haemolytic anaemia, necrosis of liver cells, gastro-intestinal bleeding, or even Reye's syndrome. The worst that could result from unfounded claims in instances of self-medication where only minor 'flu-like conditions are involved, is that the particular combination remedy may not be bought again, if it is found to be inefficacious.

Does that mean a combination such as MAP would not be available for prescription by a practitioner, unless it had undergone satisfactory clinical trials? (MAP is a combination remedy composed of three distinct moulds: mucor (from decaying vegetable matter), asperegillus (found in soil, faeces and on fruit, converting startch to fermentable sugars), and penicillium (common mildew)). It does not mean that at all, because it is not sold as a specific. A practitioner may prescribe it for a patient with a fungal condition on one occasion, or for another with seasonal hayfever, or for one with candidiasis, or for one with a dry prickly throat and an irritating cough, or for a variety of other conditions. In other words, the homoeopath is making this choice based on decisions compatible with homoeopathic practice. In that context, the practitioner's professional discretion remains inviolate. The homoeopaths, and the prescribing naturopaths, it would seem at present, need fear no restrictions in this area. They are free to decide, on the basis exemplified with the MAP, what combinations they want for their patients. This, certainly, would also include ready-made combinations.

Where, then, is the rub? What does a 6D limit actually mean? The writer's understanding of the situation, were it to become reality now, is as follows:

1. No combination remedies at all with any components under the 6D potency limit will be available to any practitioner or pharmacist, because these would not be allowed any simplified form of registration. Exorbitant licensing fees, after undergoing thorough clinical trials, which are certainly time-consuming and done at prohibitive cost, would in any event price them out of the market, since homoeopaths could effective prescribe single homoeopathic remedies in comparable combinations much more cheaply should they so wish to do. So could any orthodox medical practitioner or prescribing naturopath.

2. Single homoeopathic prescriptions in low potencies by all practitioners will remain altogether unaffected.

3. Oral and external combination remedies with all components above the 6D potency limit will be classified as 'specifics', which means they have to undergo clinical trials if they are to be sold 'over-the-counter' or by 'pharmacist's prescription', but could be offered a simplified registration procedure if they were to be available to patients on a practitioner's prescription only' basis.

Two comments are perhaps worth making here: One is that Ronald W Davey *et al* have recently published a study[4] in which, *inter alia*, tests for drug interactions (within the study's context) were undertaken on 12 monoeopathic mother tinctures in all combinations as mixtures of equal parts of any two of them. Such assays were designed to show whether the observed antibacterial effect of the two medicines in combination is additive, synergistic, antagonistic or unchanged, compared to either of them separately. It is significant that five pairs produced a clear synergistic effect, by at least doubling their cumulative effectiveness, while one pair (*Hydrastis canadensis* with *Eucalyptus globulus*) showed an antagonistic effect, whereby their joint effectiveness was half that of *Hydrastis* alone, and a quarter of *Eucalyptus* alone. In other words, it is clear that when mother tinctures, and presumably low potencies, are mixed, the effects could be quite different from those of the single constituent remedies severally. It is for this and similar reasons that the effectiveness or otherwise of low potency combinations is said to be non-deducible from the effects of its primary constituent remedies.

The other comment is that it seems very likely that the manufacturers of combination remedies will begin to change their formulae in the near future so that all components will be at or above the 6D potency level. Since the effects of one medicine at different potencies are usually startlingly different, and since there is equally no firm knowledge of the effects of remedies combined at medium or higher potencies, it will demand of the practitioners who use 'complexes' a complete familiarisation-de-novo. The effects of such newly formulated combinations, where the names of constituents may remain the same, will be that the potencies have all moved upward. It is certain that no-one will know what can be expected of such 'revised' remedies.

UK recognition of non-orthodox remedies and practices

The four principal categories of natural remedies are anthroposophic, biochemic, homoeopathic and phytotherapeutic (herbal) medicines. These four have enjoyed *de jure* recognition in the UK since 1978 when, in Statutory Instrument S141 *schedule 5*, the received special exemption status relative to advertising. This unequivocally represents official recognition in law by the UK Government of the principle of plurality of choice in medicine. Elsewhere, in paragraph 4.8 (p13) of the Department of Health and Social Security's *Medicines Act Leaflet MAL 1* (September 1984), a special exclusion of practitioners' exemptions from licensing specifically names non-orthodox practitioners, such as homoeopaths, naturopaths, etc, representing a similar recognition of the principle of plurality of choice in therapeutic approach. This recognition is rudimentary, however, when compared with some other EC member states. In France, the Securité Sociale supports the stated categories of medication to the same extent and under the same conditions as orthodox medicines. In Germany, a mature pluralism is evident in their *Medicines Act*, by which distinct state commissions are established that severally advise on anthroposophic, homoeopathic, phytotherapeutic and orthodox medicines. They are of equal rank and are fully acknowledged as experts in their field who are each free to apply their own standards. The UK has a long way to go in this aspect.

The UK Medicines Act of 1968

Whatever the final *Directive* may stipulate, it may require whole sections of the *Medicines Act* to be augmented, repealed or amended, as the case may be.

Therapeutic freedom as a basic democratic right

It may be appropriate to quote recent statements from representative sources from both the orthodox and the non-orthodox camps on this subject. First, the World Medical Association's *Statement on Access to Health Care* adopted by the 40th World Medical Assembly in Vienna in September 1988:

"Freedom of choice –

All health care delivery systems should provide each individual with the greatest possible personal freedom of choice in selecting a provider or health care mechanisms, regardless of whether they are based in the private or public sector."[5]

From the non-orthodox side it seems worth quoting Karl F Libeau, president of the Professional Association of German Naturopaths (Fachverband Deutscher Heilpraktiker e V) in his formal address on the occasion of Germany's national Heilpraktiker day this year (author's translation):

"Freedom is indivisible. If freedom as a basic attitude is to make any sense, it must be lived actively in all aspects of our lives. Freedom will not countenance enclaves of patronisation and servility. Along with economic freedom, with the freedom of opinion, with the freedom of religion, with electoral freedom, with the unhindered choice of residence and of a work place ... with personal freedom, also ranks – indispensably – therapeutic freedom."[6]

What of unresolved differences between EC Member States?

The first is a dispute between the homoeopathic pharmacists of France and Germany that has been continuing for 15 years and shows no sign of being settled. The cynics say it suits the parties to keep it unresolved, because that way the homoeopathic regulations concerning medicines cannot be finalised. After all what is a 6D, if the mother tincture remains undefined? And the dispute, of course, concerns the pharmacopoeial parameters of mother tincture preparation as these should appear in the *European Homoeopathic Pharmacopoeia*. Another unresolved issue is that many herbal, mineral, vitamin, microbiotic and amino-acid products are classed as food supplements in the UK, but are defined as medicines in many other EC countries. Could preparations be sold as food in the UK, when imported into a country in which they are considered to be medications, be blocked and possibly lead to criminal action against the importer? And would the pressures from outside inexorably drive the British Government ultimately to fall in line with the majority of Europeans?

A further issue that seems to confuse many people stems from the fact that states such as Portugal and Italy that have no legal mechanism for registering non-orthodox medicines will (in terms of *Directive SYN 251 article 6*) have to allow the sale of such medicines if these are actually registered in another EC state. (The Italian law mentioned above, of course, makes a total nonsense of this). The confusion arises when people incorrectly say this means, for example, that a remedy registered in France or Germany will thereby automatically be allowed to be sold freely in the UK, where it is not registered. Regrettably it does not mean that at all, because the UK, in fact, has its own legal mechanism for the registration of medicines. But would that mean everything registered in one country might eventually need to become registered in all the others? If it does not mean that, would not an anomaly be created identical to the one now underlying in the inter-state vitamin supplement debacle? Rumour has it that a solution may be adopted so that a medicine which has obtained rgistration in two EC member states automatically attains the status of pan-EC multi-registration. Since there are differing standards of rigorousness applied in these procedures in different countries, some manufacturers are already preparing to obtain their second registrations in countries with the laxest protocol.

The 'Four Freedoms' of the EC

The free movement of capital and goods, and of its people (and their services) are three of the EC's 'four freedoms'. The fourth is the right of establishment, meaning the freedom of any EC passport holder to carry on his/her business or professional activity in any other EC member state. There should be nothing to prevent, say, a British naturopath migrating to Italy or any other EC country to carry on the gainful activity of a naturopath, except that this is illegal in Italy. In extreme cases, he might even be jailed for doing that. So where is that 'fourth freedom' for a business, or the protected status of the professions, in the EC? It has been said with a modicum of wry justification that practitioners who are not registered with the GMC in the UK (or equivalent in another EC country) are, by turns, classified in some EC member states as running either "a business and not a professional practice", or "an illegal practice and not a business", whichever happens to be the more damning to the practitioner concerned in terms of the statutorily entrenched prejudice of the particular national authority.

The question needs to be asked again[7]: would an academic education, at least to the level of the orthodox medical practitioner, in fact, not be the one safeguard for the future of non-orthodox medicine and its practitioners?

The Government of the UK may feel obliged, in the foreseeable future, to insist on properly defined professional categories of non-orthodox practitioners, backed up by solid academic training. It may become necessary, for instance, to be able with certainty to distinguish absolutely between a lay person and a professional naturopath or homoeopath, if a 'practitioner only' prescription is to make any sense – or, for that matter, be enforceable. The alternative for practitioners may be to forego the right to prescribe certain remedies in certain potencies, or the right to prescribe at all.

Certainly some amendments to both draft *Directives* will need to be proposed in Brussels as a matter of some urgency. The situation remains very fluid and the author's mind not a little boggled by the ostrich policy pursued by many organisations representing practitioners in the UK.

References

1. Huggon T. Rule by Brussels: liberation or liquidation for natural medicines? *The Homoeopath* 1990; 10(2): 33–39. Quoting from a letter to himself (5 May 1988) from WG Robertson, Office of the Medicines Commission, UK Dept Health (p35).
2. Huggon *op cit.*
3. On 17th June 1948 the American Institute of Homoeopathy, which in this country is often taken to represent the classical tradition, surprisingly approved a resolution, which it, moreover, fully re-affirmed on 11th February 1981, and which has been officially incorporated into the *Homoeopathic Pharmacopoeia* of the United States, *vide* Supplement A-1982, page 76.
4. Davey RW, McGregor JA, Grange JM. Screening tests

for antibacterial substances in plant extracts. *Comp Med Res* 1990; 4(1): 1–7.

5. Editorial. World Medical Association Statement on Access to Health Care: adopted by the 40th World Medical Assembly, Vienna, Austria, September 1988. *World Med J* 1989; 36(3): 42–43.

6. Liebau KF. Ansprache von DH-Praesident. *Der Heilpraktiker* 1990; 36(8): 61–64.

7. Gaier HC. Implementation of resolute educational strategy: essential element to secure the future for non-orthodox medicine. *Comp Med Res* 1989; 3(2): 30–35.

Index